M

"Remarkable . . . Com earing insight into the battle to stay a nd humor and a radiant courage."
—Ted Koppel

"[A] compelling memoir . . . Silverstein's humor and devotion to her husband and son see her through, and by the end you'll be rooting for her next twenty years." —Kim Hubbard, *People* (3 of 4 stars)

"A grueling, ultimately uplifting story of endurance."
—Kristin Kloberdanz, *Chicago Tribune*

"Truly compelling, *Sick Girl* sucked me in from the get go. Amy Silverstein's story is amazing and inspiring." —Mary Roach

"Read this and promise us you'll never whine about having a cold again." —Colleen Oakley, *Marie Claire*

"[A] mesmeric human drama of living life as a heart transplant recipient . . . A superb writer with a wry, biting sense of humor . . . Silverstein is a natural raconteur with a story so compelling readers won't want to put this book down." —Maura Sostack, *Library Journal* (starred review)

"Silverstein is an inspired storyteller. Her engaging language and sharp insight make *Sick Girl* both compelling and moving. Few of us undergo a heart transplant at twenty-four, but we can recognize our own stories in this incisive, unflinching look at life, love, and extraordinary courage." —Susan Cheever

"[*Sick Girl*] is frank and honest and spares no one."
—Ian Munro, *Sydney Morning Herald*

"Sets the record straight about a so-called medical miracle."
—*Kirkus Reviews*

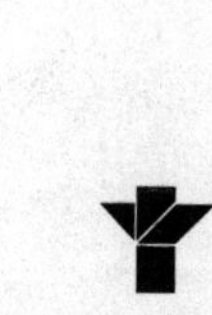

Sick Girl

Author's Note

Out of respect for the privacy of people who appear in this book, I have changed their names and some physical descriptions.

SICK GIRL

Amy Silverstein

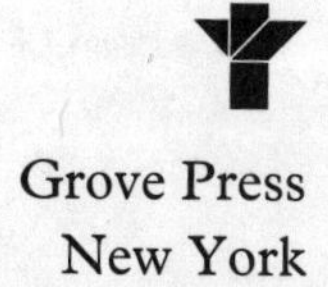

Grove Press
New York

Published simultaneously in Canada
Printed in the United States of America

FIRST PAPERBACK EDITION

ISBN-10: 0-8021-4387-3
ISBN-13: 978-0-8021-4387-7

Grove Press
an imprint of Grove/Atlantic, Inc.
841 Broadway
New York, NY 10003

Distributed by Publishers Group West

www.groveatlantic.com

08 09 10 11 12 10 9 8 7 6 5 4 3 2 1

For Scott and Casey
– my air –

A man who becomes conscious of the responsibility he bears toward a human being who affectionately waits for him, or to an unfinished work, will never be able to throw away his life. He knows the "why" for his existence and will be able to bear almost any "how."

—Viktor Frankl

How little it takes to make life unbearable: a pebble in the shoe, a cockroach in the spaghetti, a woman's laugh.

—H. L. Mencken

Sick Girl

Pre-Game

As I stand here counting out three pairs of underwear and four pairs of socks, I think of the little boy who will reach into his suitcase and find them waiting there for him—as if by magic—along with everything else he might need this weekend. I thank the slow passage of time for keeping this son of mine young enough still to see the world as a seamless sleight of hand: a quarter behind the ear, the tooth fairy's dollar, a perfectly packed bag that appears out of nowhere. He doesn't yet need to know the trickery behind the wonders that come his way. He doesn't need to know how hard it is for his mother to stand here packing this bag: how tired she feels. How sick.

Today I create an illusion with a suitcase. On another day, perhaps, I might draw upon my famous French toast. I am the mother behind the curtain, after all. My son is my constant audience.

And thank goodness my hand is still quicker than his eye. I'll be sure to pack a book and a deck of cards, grape-scented kids' shampoo and a rain poncho—just in case. I will think of everything so this ten-year-old boy will be free to think of nothing: not my life expectancy, which ran out eight years ago, nor the handful of big-gun medicines I took this morning that forced me to the floor, a mommy-ball of nausea curled up on a damp bathroom rug. No, there will not be any trace of my heart transplant in the suitcase I pack for my son today.

I'm one hell of a great magician.

Hey, I think I'll toss in this mini-checkers set for the long plane ride. . . .

Almost ready to zip the bag closed now, I fold his favorite football jersey with care, running my hands over the mesh material he calls "my holy shirt," and place it neatly on top of the pile. My son is leaving for the Super Bowl with his dad tomorrow morning. Lucky kid.

I imagine them at the game sitting side by side, one pair of high knees next to one pair of low. Father and son in caps with matching football team logos, gazing ahead, rapt. The boy looks up at the man and smiles, sunlight glinting across soft bangs. The father smiles back. A memory is created.

And while this is happening there will be a woman hundreds of miles away who can't catch her breath; she will not have taken her medicine while they were away and now her body has turned against itself, just as she knew it would. Her limbs feel impossibly heavy and there is no use trying to hold them up any longer; she must give in. This mother, this wife—this reluctant survivor—has made sure to leave herself no other choice this time; there will be no saving her. She can lie down on her bedroom floor in contented resignation.

Now I don't have to try anymore, she will whisper into the carpeting beneath her cheek. *I don't have to be a goddamn miracle.*

She will close her eyes for the last time—in peace.

There will be no loving greeting for the returning football fans. There will be a death.

Can I really do this?

Maybe.

I put my son's toothbrush in a plastic bag and place it in the small suitcase with the rest of his things. My feet carry me through the house now, but I feel I am floating, lost in thought. I pass by the family room, turn back, and peek inside the door; Scott still has not gotten up from the couch. He dropped himself there about an hour ago after driving home from our appointment at the hospital. The TV is off. There is no newspaper on his lap. He hasn't even called the office to find out if anything important went on in his absence this afternoon. Seeing him like this, I feel my stomach tighten with guilt and remorse: The man I love most in the world has chosen to sit alone in tormented silence, and here I stand ten feet away from him with no idea how to break it.

I am the cause of it.

Lingering at the doorway, I watch him for a moment and then continue down the hall, furious with my heart-transplant body for coming between us again. Seventeen years of circles around my health problems have not given us any sense of resolution. The illnesses continue to come in waves, and we find ourselves caught up in an undertow that pulls us both into a fight for my life that feels more and more compulsory as time goes by. And while Scott continues to fight on, unhesitant, for me there is no longer anything natural or automatic about it. Staying alive in this body has become an obligation for me that continually raises the question of why. Why continue in a perpetual lifesaving marathon when there is no possibility of a happy, healthy end?

The answer to this question appears to me only in blurry glimpses from time to time—mostly in the calm short breaks between illnesses. Standing in my kitchen today, with my fingers curled around the handle of my son's Super Bowl suitcase, I am keenly aware that some people might say I hold the clear answer right here, right now, in the grip of my hand: the why for my continued fight for life could be—should be—my son.

Or my husband—the man who is, I'm certain, the real cause behind the apparent miracle of my continued survival. The constancy of his love and the effects it has had on my longevity should be enough to keep me fighting forever. That's what people expect from me, I know. Which is why what happened at the doctor's today is such a sorry surprise: that I would hesitate before reaching out for another buoyant, gleaming white lifesaver tossed into the perilous riptide of my heart-transplant life.

That I might not reach for it at all.

Oh, I'd have to be a crazy person to do that. Or awfully selfish. I'd be called an ungrateful organ recipient. A bad patient. A bad mother.

A hurtful, unloving wife.

I place the suitcase by the kitchen door and take a seat on the wooden bench beside it. With my hands cradling the top of my head, I pull my neck forward and let my face come down until I am looking at the floor between my feet. I notice Scott's worn-out pair of running sneakers peeking out from under the bench. Lined up just next to them is my own pair, even more battered. Seeing the evidence of our morning jogs aligned so closely this way, it strikes me for the first time how odd it is that Scott and I never go running together. From time to time he has asked me to join him, but I always say no, thanks, "I like to do my own thing," which is only partly a lie. I certainly do my own thing, but there is nothing about it that I like. Running miles with this transplanted heart is hell for me.

So is packing this suitcase.

"I'm done with Casey's bag," I say. "He's all set to go." I've made my way back down the hall to the family room again and find Scott still there, still motionless on the couch. I'm hoping to rouse him with news of the motherly chore I've just accomplished. But I know that in the eyes of my husband a well-packed suitcase is not a remarkable achievement. Not even for his heart-transplant wife—the one behind the curtain who makes everything she does look so damn easy.

How can I expect him to applaud effort that he cannot imagine?

I lift Scott's legs up a bit and move them to the inside of the couch so I can sit down next to him. My eyes rest somewhere around his knees for now. I will not look up at his face until I get the all clear: a touch on the shoulder or an invitation like, "You know I love you, but—" I need some sign that Scott isn't irreparably angry at me in spite of how I failed him today.

He lifts his hand off the couch and brings it down with a thump. "You were totally out of line with Dr. Davis. You yelled at him—at your transplant doctor. The man who has kept you alive all these years. He doesn't deserve your anger . . . and he sure doesn't deserve to hear your suicide threats."

"They're not threats," I say, keeping my eyes down.

"If you remember correctly, I set up the appointment for today. I called Dr. Davis. And he was nice enough to sit down with both of us—for over an hour—to work this thing out. Find a way to make your life more livable. But you attacked him like it was his fault. And then you tell him—and me—that you're going to stop taking your transplant medicines. How is he supposed to react? I mean, come on. What do you want him to say?"

I'm not sure how to answer this. The truth is, I'd like to hear Dr. Davis say that it's really okay with him if I go now—that I've done an amazing job in this body and that I've withstood more than any one person should. I'd like to hear him agree with what I've said all along: my life was not really saved back when I was just a twenty-four-year-old law student with a virus in her heart—no, my life was taken away by this heart transplant and I can't expect to ever have it back, not even a small slice of it. I'd want him to say that he is proud of me for hanging on for seventeen years: with two strong hands, with bite, and with effort, intelligence, and an appearance of normalcy that have been astounding. I'd want Dr. Davis to honor me and let me go.

But instead, I tell Scott, "I don't know what I want him to say."

"Well, then, what am *I* supposed to say? When I ask your doctor to meet with us and then you dump all over him. When I hear you go off about how you won't take your medicine. How do you think *I* feel?"

"It must be awful."

The words sound flimsy, even to me.

"Do you realize that since this whole post-transplant lymphoma thing came up last week, you must've said to me ten times that you want to end your life? And I listen to you. Then there are hugs and more listening. We spend a lot of time talking about it. And you're still saying that you want to give up and die. I schedule an appointment with your doctor. I'm supportive. I'm there for you. But the sadness, the anger, the suicide talk—they just keep coming. There's no end. It just goes on and on and on. . . ."

That's why he feels frustrated and fed up, he says; it's not so much the nature of my complaint (Scott says he understands how a cancer threat, in addition to my heart transplant, can force me to the very end of my rope), rather, it's the endlessness of it that wrecks him. He needs a break from my anguish—or at least from the way I express it and how often.

I tell Scott, though I'm not sure he believes me, that I truly want to give him the break he deserves. I want to make things easier for him.

The suitcase, for instance. I packed it so he wouldn't have to. I don't tell him that my heartbeat felt terribly wrong the whole time I did it. I keep from him the details of the crippling nausea I felt; the trembling hands that challenged me to button and fold my son's shirt without breaking into tears. But I know Scott is not interested in suitcases. He wants an end.

So do I. We just see this end differently. Scott would like to see the end of my despair; I want to end my suffering. They are not the same wish.

I lift my eyes now and look into Scott's for the first time since I sat down beside him on the couch. He looks back at me through a haze of weariness. Self-blame rises up in me: I haven't spared him enough; I haven't thought of him enough; I haven't kept enough of my heart-transplant self behind the curtain.

Or maybe I've kept too much of me there. Perhaps there is a price to be paid for hiding the truth about how I live in this body, and I am paying it now: being misunderstood.

My family will leave for the Super Bowl tomorrow morning. They will go on my insistence; I would not allow an acute flare-up of my medical problems to hold them back. Scott bought these game tickets months ago, after all. Casey has been counting the days. And besides, I don't feel especially sick or weak. I jogged this morning: a nod to Scott that I'm bouncing back from the crisis that culminated in the showdown with Dr. Davis, and that it is okay to leave me.

Bathed in the green light I have given him, Scott will wake to an early alarm clock, walk down the hall to our son's room, and find him there, already up. Casey will spring from the bed, throwing the covers away from his body in one swift move. Then he'll soar down the stairs, taking three at a time—in his pajamas.

Scott will have to call out and remind him to put some clothes on.

Right! Clothes!

Then there will be a few moments of commotion as father and son begin rummaging through drawers. Scott will pull out a pair of pants that are too small. Casey will grab a sweater that is way too warm for where they're headed. Then, in the same moment, they'll turn their heads and notice the jeans, T-shirt, underwear, socks, and lightweight zip-up sweatshirt folded neatly on the chair. A grin will come up between them as they realize, in silence:

It was Amy.

It was Mom.

And I bet she packed my suitcase too.

Of course I did. But I'm not sure if I will be here to unpack it as well.

Over this Super Bowl weekend, I will spend a lot of time thinking about endings. And beginnings and middles. Heart viruses, hospitals, and being saved. Bravery and hope. Reluctance and resignation.

And responsibility: to a son, a well-meaning doctor, and a husband who must be some kind of angel.

Love is exhausting.

1

My heart transplant was there in the lines of my father's palm. Madame Clara saw it right away. She was not just another fortune-teller with a shack along the Atlantic City boardwalk; Madame Clara was a gifted seer (or so her sign said). She knew that a man like my father, middle aged with a fine leather belt and Gucci shoes, along with my stepmother, Beverly, a well-kept blonde with country-club good looks, would be likely to doubt her psychic advice even as they sought it. They were casual drop-ins: the kind of customers who wander in on a lark, husband pushing wife or vice versa, with a playful nudge. "Aw, come on. . . . It'll be fun." If people like this were ever going to take her seriously, Madame Clara figured they would have to be eased into believing. She'd first have to dazzle my father and Beverly with some facts, things only a true fortune-teller could read in the crisscross lines and intricate folds on the underside of my father's right hand.

"You are in a family business. There is stock involved," she said, offering up the first evidence of her clairvoyance.

"Well, you got me there. Score one for the great Madame Clara!" My father was in a playful mood as usual, ready to challenge the dark-haired woman sitting opposite him with fast quips and charming good humor. "Seems you know me like the back of your hand—or my hand, as the case may be."

She continued intently, her black eyes unwavering. “You have an important deal in the making; it will fall through. Do not feel distressed when this happens. Something bigger awaits you.”

“Bigger than a bread box?”

Madame Clara laid her pointer finger on the center of my father’s palm and traced a diagonal line slowly, stopping at points to whisper their significance. “Respect. The rewards of hard work. Bounty.”

“Await me, right?”

She looked up from his hand. “Yes, but only after a disappointment. You will not get what you have been seeking.”

These words had significance for my father. The year was 1984. He was in the process of trying to sell the family business that his father and uncles had started some forty-five years earlier, which had grown to become a publicly traded company on the Stock Exchange. On the day my father offered his palm to a fortune-teller for the first time in his life, he believed he held in his pocket a firm offer from a large conglomerate to buy the business for a share price that was more than respectable. It was an imminent coup; the company had fallen on hard times and my father was one of the major forces to save it with some tough decisions and careful maneuvers. He was not a popular manager at first, but his efforts breathed not only life but unprecedented productivity into the company. To pull off a sale at this point would yield a profit for shareholders, including the cousins he’d sent out the door.

Did Madame Clara just tell him that the deal would fall through?

My father grimaced.

“Oh, Arthur, don’t be ridiculous,” Beverly said. The sudden furrow in my father’s brow told his wife just what he was thinking. She grabbed his forearm and gave it a little shake, followed by a couple of reassuring pats. “Well, for Pete’s sake, there must be something else in that hand of his, Madame—ah . . . Clara?" She forced herself into a grin but there was nothing cheerful about it; Beverly's expression was flat-out imploring.

It was time to change the subject, and Madame Clara was ready. She had been holding back but would now reveal the prophecy she may have seen and had been reluctant to mention: that one of my father's two daughters would become very sick.

My father had not told her he had any children at all, let alone two daughters; the fortune-teller had hit upon another truth. There was Jodie, who'd just graduated from college, and her younger sister, Amy, who still had two years to go. Both were healthy young women.

"There will be a surgery—a serious one. And a miraculous recovery. The daughter will be okay."

"Splendid," my father said. "Next time, let's stick to the collapse of my business deals. It's more fun."

Madame Clara shrugged. "I see what I see—dark and light."

"Maybe I should have washed my hands first," he said. My father reached into his pocket for a twenty dollar bill and handed it to Madame Clara with a wink. "Thanks for the memories!"

Or at least that's how I pictured it. My father had recounted his fortune-teller story so many times it ran like a movie in my head. The first time I heard it, Madame Clara's prophecy about the sale of the family business had already come true: the original deal had fallen through just as she said it would, only to be replaced several months later with a different buyout arrangement for nearly double the price. Dark and light—that's what she'd told him. Oh, she was right. Madame Clara was the real McCoy. What a story!

And what a nightmare: there had also been a prediction about an illness. My father had to keep this part quiet and hope with every bit of the skeptic still left in him that it would not come true. But the amazing Madame Clara had turned him into something of a believer. The best my father could do was push the sick daughter prediction to the back of his mind, stay silent about it, and wait for the passage of time to prove that the fortune-teller's insights had been imperfect.

Three years later, illness hit me hard and fast; I would undergo the serious surgery that Madame Clara had foreseen. My sister, Jodie, would remain healthy. In time, I would move on to a recovery that was every bit the miracle that had shown up in my father's palm. But the fortune-teller had also said that I, the sick daughter, would be okay; this part of her prediction was flawed. While I would, in fact, survive for a surprisingly long time after surgery, nothing about living with a fragile heart would ever be okay with me. This is not to say that Madame Clara was wrong. She was, after all, reading my father's palm, not mine, so whatever she drew from it would naturally reflect his perceptions and experiences to come. My father, like nearly everyone else in my life, would always see me as okay in my post-surgery body. Perhaps Madame Clara had not misread his future at all.

But she'd misread mine. Months before I would sense the first inkling of a heart problem, I took a short trip to Atlantic City with my boyfriend, Scott. On my suggestion, we sought out Madame Clara's shack on the boardwalk and there it was, right where my father said it would be. Scott was reluctant to go in. The whole fortune-telling thing gave him the creeps, he said, even while parting the glass beads that served as the door to the reading room. As Scott took his first tentative step inside, I reached down and pinched his butt cheek, hard and quick. Into the air he flew, with a gasp.

"And I didn't even have to yell *boo!*" I teased.

"I'll show you *boo!*" He spun around and grabbed the sides of my waist, squeezing in spurts that brought me to breathless laughter within seconds.

Madame Clara emerged from behind a makeshift curtain and sat, annoyed, behind her crystal ball. I squirmed out from Scott's clutches and brought the fun to an end, knowing I was in the presence of the great seer who'd predicted, with amazing precision, the fate of my family's business. It excited me to think of what she might say about my own destiny; I'd just finished my first year of law school at NYU, and I was in love—real love—for the first time.

I offered up my palm. This had to be good.

Madame Clara fell silent. Her eyes went soft and out of focus, almost as if she were refusing to look closely into my hand.

I felt the urge to help her along. "Um . . . will I have children?"

"I see four," she said.

"What about health?"

She turned my hand over and patted the top of it. "Health looks good. You will live a long life."

This was the end of my reading with Madame Clara. She charged me only five dollars; it lasted less than three minutes. Scott kept his palm to himself.

A good fortune-teller is focused on the hand in front of her. Hands contain lines; they are simple to read. But faces—especially young attractive ones—are more complex. And when they're attached to lean, youthful, unblemished bodies, faces can be misleading. Even obscuring.

The diagnosis of my illness might have come about differently had my family doctor studied a little palmistry. Or maybe if he'd closed his eyes and just listened to what I was telling him instead of being blindsided by the pretty first-year law student sitting on the exam table wearing nothing but a light blue hospital gown. It does not take tremendous beauty to throw an Ivy League–educated physician off the scent of a menacing illness. It's the coming together of circumstances that will do it—with or without a mane of long wavy hair and a perky bosom. Take an admittedly studious, overachieving twenty-three-year-old woman at a highly competitive law school; give her tightness in the chest and a couple of episodes of passing out; send her to the doctor's office, cheerful and bright-eyed, with a bounce in her step; and have her giggling at his jokes and at the first touch of the cold stethoscope on her back. Together, these can be enough to make any doctor assume, at first blush, that there is nothing terribly wrong with this young woman.

Dr. Clark gave me the obligatory exam. He looked into my eyes with a light and my ears with a scope. He asked me to touch my nose and walk in a straight line. Then, after listening to my heart for a few seconds, he mentioned casually that he'd heard a slight clicking that I "might want to get checked out sometime." He was thinking mitral valve prolapse, a generally benign condition that could possibly explain the sound he'd heard. Then he took my blood pressure; his eyebrows shot up almost to his hairline. "Wow, that's low!" he said.

"Too low?"

"Aw . . . what's too low?"

I didn't know what was too low. That's why I was asking.

"Could it be why I've been passing out?"

"Sure! You should salt your food. Lots of salt. Salt it all, if you like." He told me I should consider myself lucky to be one of the people who didn't have to feel guilty when they reached for the salt shaker. Dr. Clark was an old pro at seeing the bright side.

Later, in his office, with me now dressed in my street clothes and sitting opposite him across a paper-ridden desk, my doctor pronounced me well, saying he couldn't find anything wrong except the low blood pressure. The stresses of law school were getting to me, he said. That's all it was. He gave me an empathetic "It's tough the first year, isn't it?" followed by "But not too tough for a girl like you, I bet!" Then, just before I slipped out the door, Dr. Clark held his arms out to me, just as he did for all his patients, and I knew I was in for one of his signature bear hugs, with that barrel chest of his so solid against me it hardly seemed to yield at all to the pressure of body against body. His hugs had been taking my family's breath away for years; and today especially I was glad to have the familiar comforts of Dr. Clark so close by—at New York Hospital, just a fifteen-minute cab ride from my law dorm at NYU.

On my way back downtown I bought a large blue container of Morton's salt and poured a good-sized mound of iodized blood pressure lifter into my palm. I licked it off in one swipe; I really didn't want to pass out again. But I did pass out again. And again—in the shower, waiting for an elevator, brushing my hair by the mirror. I didn't call Dr. Clark to tell him his salt cure was not working for me, and I never went to have that little click checked out either—not even after I started vomiting blood. I felt at fault for these body symptoms and was embarrassed that I couldn't bring my stress level down to the point where they would just disappear. Dr. Clark had told me I was healthy, right? I could only blame myself for not feeling well. *Nervous law student. Must calm down. Eat salt.*

I would look back on the early stages of my illness and wonder how many other young women had ever stared into a toilet bowl full of their own blood-streaked vomit, flushed it down, and dashed off to a two-hour seminar in Constitutional Law. Probably none. My brushing aside of symptoms was uniquely stupid. There must have been something—*what was it, what was it?*—that led me to ignore the obvious. Only in retrospect would I recognize that it was youth, coupled with the absence of serious childhood illness, that could dull down the medical-danger radar in a girl to the point where peril hardly registered at all. Add to this an obliging physician with the same defective detection system, plus a penchant for the jolly, and what you've got is a recipe for massive denial that cooks up into a ticking time bomb.

Back in Dr. Clark's office one year later, I would find my blind optimism blown to bits. This time my symptoms were different and more serious: I couldn't breathe. But strangely enough this was not the main focus of my complaint. It was more my chest that was the problem, or so I believed. It felt heavy and uncomfortably full, as if

I'd eaten three years worth of Thanksgiving dinners in one sitting. I told Dr. Clark that there seemed to be something wrong with my stomach; food didn't want to go down. It felt worse at night when I lay in bed. I'd even heard a gurgling deep down in the center of my chest—like there was water in there or something. "My digestion isn't right. I feel it here," I said, placing my hand over my left breast without the faintest appearance of worry. There was nothing about my twenty-four-year-old life that would prompt me to make a connection between the location of my hand and the heart that lay beneath it.

The heaviness in my chest turned out to be due not to poor digestion, as I'd thought, but rather to a grossly enlarged heart that was literally bursting out of me. And the gurgling sound I'd heard? That was water in my lungs. I'd been listening to it night after night as I lay in bed, a crackling that came with each exhalation; it didn't scare me at all. I figured it must be part of that food "caught in my pipe." Such simple words and innocent explanations came naturally from a young woman who hadn't been sick since her childhood ear infections. I was understandably naïve. My medical vocabulary was nonexistent and my self-diagnostic skills immature. Pipes and stomach trouble—that was the best I could come up with. My imagination could only go so far as a bellyache.

But Dr. Clark was probably able to conjure up a range of possibilities—and perhaps one horrifying probability—from the obvious severity of my symptoms. A quick step up on his scale showed I had gained eight pounds since weighing myself at home two days earlier (a sure sign that my body did not have the strength to expel water as it should). A blood-pressure check proved that a whole year of salting my food hadn't helped my numbers to rise one bit. An external palpation of my abdomen was normal except for one troubling discovery that had nothing at all to do with my digestive system: I wasn't able to catch my breath while lying down on the exam table. Even before he put his stethoscope to my chest,

Dr. Clark had an idea of what he was dealing with, although he could hardly believe it. From what he'd seen so far, the young woman on his exam table seemed to have congestive heart failure, a disease found mostly in the elderly or in middle-aged people who'd suffered several heart attacks. A diagnosis of this disease usually meant that at least some portion of vital heart muscle had been damaged beyond repair.

The cause of this damage varied case to case in congestive-heart-failure patients. Dr. Clark could not imagine what might have been the cause of mine, but at the moment it didn't matter: left untreated, congestive heart failure could be fatal.

It must not have been easy for him to put his dark suspicions to the final test. "Let's take a listen," he said.

I opened the front of my hospital gown and lifted my chin into the air. Dr. Clark leaned his head toward me as he concentrated on the sound of my heartbeat. It didn't take long for him to realize that the little click he'd heard only one year earlier had turned into an ominous thud. Instead of the bright sounds doctors typically hear when listening to a healthy heartbeat, there were gallops—spurts of effort followed by a run of chaotic aftershocks—and then a short period of tortured lumbering. Dr. Clark knew he had just listened in on a sick heartbeat that was out of his league as a general internist. "Why don't you get dressed and meet me in my office. We'll talk, okay?" he said, without a hint of anxiety. It was important not to get me upset or excited—not with the way my heart was beating today.

When I walked into Dr. Clark's office he was already on the phone. He smiled and gestured for me to take a seat. After finishing one phone call he immediately went on to the next and then the next. Each time he brought the receiver to his ear, he'd hold up a finger to let me know that he would be just one more minute; just one more phone call and then I'd get that talk I'd been promised. I looked on as Dr. Clark reached up again and again to rub the back of his neck, beginning each new phone call with an audible exhalation and a plea: "Can you do me a favor here?" He was trying to arrange for me to have tests done immediately, even though it was past five on a Friday night.

"There, now we've got it," he said, handing me a sheet of paper with locations and times written on it. "I need you to go do these tests for me, if you would."

"Tonight? Now?"

"If you would, please. I just want to check a few things out, okay? Go now, dear. Come back and see me when you're done. I'll wait here in the office for you."

"But won't it be late? It's Friday night."

"Doesn't bother me a bit; I have a lot of paperwork to tackle. Don't worry yourself about me."

"All right, as long as you don't mind," I said, gathering my things together and heading for the door. I thought it was awfully nice of Dr. Clark to hang around just for my stomach problem.

"Some of these testing places are a couple of blocks away from here. You'll have to do a fair amount of buzzing around. So please, dear . . . walk slowly."

I lingered beneath the door frame for a moment. "Sure, okay," I said.

I did not notice until after I'd spun through the revolving doors of the hospital and out onto the street that I had left Dr. Clark's office without a big bear hug. He'd remained seated for the first time ever, elbows on the desk, fingers massaging both his temples. I thought I saw him reach for the phone again as I walked out.

My visit with Madame Clara predated the fateful appointment with Dr. Clark by just three months. I'd chosen to ask the fortune-teller about my health—a question that might have seemed odd coming from a young woman. But even back then, during my short weekend trip to Atlantic City with my boyfriend, I had a sense that I was not well. I'd been sitting with Scott at dinner in some casino restaurant in Caesar's Palace, maroon velvet walls all around us and huge silver goblets on the table as symbols of a tacky Ancient Rome. A photographer dressed in a bedsheet toga wandered over and asked if he could take our picture. I wished that he'd skipped our table; nausea and light-headedness occupied my attention, and the last thing I wanted to do was strike a pretty pose. Scott did not know this, of course, and asked for one photo—of me, alone on my side of the booth—so he could have a memory shot for his wallet. We'd only been dating two months, but Scott already knew I was more than a little bit camera shy and would have to be coaxed into a smile. As the photographer stepped backward from the table and toyed with his lens, Scott leaned across and whispered to me in an accent he couldn't have intended to come off so comically French, "You are my leetle Rom-an godd-ess! Your beauty could fill ze Coliseum!" I laughed, my chin resting on my palm, elbow on the table, and—*click*—the photographer caught me in a full smile. It was a pose Scott would carry in his wallet for the next seventeen years: his lighthearted Roman goddess always there at his fingertips, twinkle-eyed and lovely. He saw only happiness in the photo, but for me the image contained a painful memory; I had been concealing something from Scott that night. Even as I laughed at his comparing my beauty to a Roman sculpture, my mind was troubled: *I really don't feel well. This is something bad and I know it.*

A haunting memory of the photograph came to mind as a car whisked me up First Avenue to my first-ever appointment with a cardiologist. I began searching my mind for signs that I'd missed or had ignored over the last year, ones that might have been responsible for landing me in the backseat of this car. I felt proud at first, for having been so courageous through months of symptoms that might have sent a weaker woman running back to the doctor who'd waved her good-bye with a hug and a saltshaker prescription. But then I thought myself a fool who just might have kidded her way straight into a medical emergency. As the city blocks rushed by and blurred, negativity and doubt began to set in. I shivered with regret and shame, recalling how I'd put my faith in a container of Morton's salt. Deep down, I hadn't fully believed Dr. Clark at the time he'd said it would cure my low-blood-pressure problem, but I'd found his jaunty prescription hard to resist and his bear hug reassuring.

The Friday-night circuit of diagnostic tests he ordered had revealed an unspecified something wrong with my heart; by Monday I had an appointment with a cardiac specialist, Dr. Daniel Bradley. My father and Beverly, as my parents, were the natural choice for driving and accompanying me. I would have liked for Scott to be with me as well today, but he was hours away at Penn Law School, caught up in hours of classes and a part-time job, so I'd told him to stay put; I was fine and would speak with him afterward. I'd also considered asking my sister to come but then thought better of it; Jodie was severely doctor- and hospital-phobic, averse to the point of true hysteria when faced with white coats and syringes (even when aimed at someone else). Her presence would only have added to the fear and anger that had been mounting inside me.

By the time my parents' car stopped in front of the medical building, I had worked up a huff of angry disappointment that radiated far beyond the confines of Dr. Clark's office and my own foolish denial. I was already irritated at my future cardiologist, Dr. Bradley, and I hadn't even met him yet. I was also plenty leery. Thirty blocks northbound in my father's car had given me enough time to arrive at a troubling conclusion: doctors cannot be trusted; they make awful, awful mistakes.

My father and Beverly, though, would keep the faith and hold fast to the idea of super-doctors, with Dr. Clark being the most illustrious among them. By extension, Dr. Bradley was raised high in their esteem for having been his top cardiologist pick. Were it not for Marvin (Dr. Clark's first name rolled off my father's tongue as if he were referring to a golfing buddy), it would have taken weeks to land an appointment with a cardiologist of such renown. My father insisted I was fortunate: Marvin was there when we needed him, with his sharp diagnostic skills and unparalleled web of best-doctor connections.

Lucky me. Lucky us.

"But he got it wrong," I said, surprising my father. I hadn't yet detailed for him the progression of my office visits with Dr. Clark, because up until this point it hadn't seemed important. But now that my father was expecting me to worship this new cardiologist as a blessed offshoot of our family internist, I felt compelled to speak up and put both merely mortal physicians in proper perspective: neither one of them deserved our blind devotion.

My father appeared not to have heard what I just said—or else he was pretending real hard.

"I went to see Dr. Clark last year because I was passing out a lot. He said it was just low blood pressure. Obviously he was wrong."

"Come on, honey, did you tell him you were passing out? Did you? Really, did you actually tell him?" This was Beverly talking. She turned her head to glance back at me from the passenger's seat and threw off that high-eyebrow mother glare of hers, accusatory and questioning at the same time. It was a look she'd been flashing my way since I was eight years old, perhaps because Beverly understood that young girls needed to be on the receiving end of this kind of lingering stare from time to time. It was a sign of love. Beverly knew I had never gotten much in the way of affectionate maternal scorn at home. My parents' divorce had left me at age five with a mother who wouldn't bother expending the effort it would take to raise an eyebrow for my benefit; she was too busy fawning over a glass of scotch—and then another and another. I had begun mixing my mother's drinks on request in the second grade; a hair-raising howl would float up to my room, and quickly as I could drop a Magic Marker in my lap, I would be down in the drinking den with the red-haired terror I was forced to call Mom. I'd count out three ice cubes into her favorite glass and then douse them with Johnnie Walker, poured to the level that matched the length of my ink-stained thumb.

This would all continue until it was time for me to go to college, at which point I left my bartending duties behind forever, along with the face, voice, and liquor-soaked rages of the exacting patron in the hell-pit cocktail bar that was my childhood home. I didn't look back. Didn't call. Didn't write. Didn't share my college academic awards, my law-school admission, or even my heart illness. It seemed to me I hadn't lost much by running off this way; all I had really given up was a mother in the most attenuated sense. It was Beverly who had truly raised me and Jodie since little girlhood, taking root as a nurturing presence in our lives—if only on weekends and school holidays, according to my father's rights under the divorce agreement. In between visits, there were frequent conversations on the phone. Beverly showered us with attention, doling out love, guidance, and advice wherever Jodie or I ran short.

And today, in the midst of a tense car-ride discussion, I would accept Beverly's insistent prodding begrudgingly, even as part of me was glad to be needled with so much interest and caring.

"Of course I told him." It was a perfect place to throw in an eyeball roll, and so I did, with drama; it was the kind of roll a mother might expect from a daughter like me.

"Maybe you should have been more insistent," she said.

"I told him what I was feeling. That's all I had to do. Dr. Clark was supposed to figure it out from there."

"And he did . . . eventually. We're lucky he caught it, I tell you. So lucky."

I slid across the backseat and out into the hard cold rain. My father and Beverly managed to make their way from car to doorway before I did because they ran like mad. At first I set out to jog the thirty feet along with them, but my strength gave out and I couldn't catch my breath. Then I remembered what Dr. Clark had told me Friday about walking slowly, and it all began to sink in: the pelting rain, the cardiologist appointment, the horror and strange humiliation of watching my father and Beverly, both nearly sixty years old, make it inside a full twenty seconds before I could. They watched with patient smiles as I slow-stepped toward them through sheets of rain, wincing. It was in this moment that I experienced for the first time in my life what it was like to be disempowered by illness; I was not able to move as fast as I wanted or needed—my twenty-four-year-old body wouldn't let me—and if I pushed through limitations with my usual stubborn strength, I feared it might cause my heart to give out. How terrifying even to think it: that I could die while trying to save myself from getting sopped by this rain! Thirty feet of distance from car to doorway appeared before me like a life-and-death choice. It was the first choice of this kind that I'd been forced to make in my life; it would not be the last.

It seemed I was caught in a rainstorm full of lessons: a momentous mind-altering downpour that would teach me with a slow, soggy trek up the steps of a medical building that youth is no protection from illness. It would also remind me—forever—that extreme weather can be an omen (for me, at least). Whenever I woke again to the sound of rain splattering sideways against my bedroom window, I would sense a portent of bad news to come. It was all I needed to set off on a slide—down, down—to a place of worry and fear about my body. I'd drop like a shot, ending at a black bottom no healthy person would ever understand, trembling beneath my quilt in secret panic.

I'm dying again. I'm dying again.

"Who wants to hear a joke?" My father was ready, as always, to distract with humor, pulling my attention away from this waiting room of cardiology patients three times my age.

"Sure, Dad, lay it on me," I said, leaning closer to him.

"A doctor finishes examining this guy and says, 'Look, I've got bad news and good news. Which one do you want first?' The guy tells him he wants the bad. 'Okay, you've got two weeks to live. I'm so sorry.' Then the guy asks what the good news could possibly be, and the doctor answers, 'See that blonde nurse down the hall there, the one with the big boobs? I'm fucking her.'"

Good one, Dad.

My father always managed to get a laugh out of me, even with the crudest and most offensive jokes. He had a gift for lighthearted delivery and a comic sense that never failed—not even in a cardiologist's waiting room.

Looking at my father's face as the smile faded from his lips, I saw nothing in his expression but easy confidence, as if he were sitting with Beverly and me in a nice restaurant waiting for our menus to arrive. Maybe it was just optimism, or maybe a worried father's denial all dressed up to achieve that casual appearance. But it was his ability to hold on to this nonchalance *after* our appointment that seemed to me most ludicrous. My father would tell me the details of a phone call he received later on from a friend, who'd reacted to my bad news by saying, "Gee, Arthur, that must've been a terrible day for you." My father had told him, yes indeed it was a horrible day—for his stock portfolio.

It so happened that my appointment with Dr. Bradley fell on October 17, 1987—also known as Black Monday—the day when the stock market went wildly bad and took a giant nosedive. It was a downfall reminiscent of the crash that set off the Great Depression. As stockbrokers and securities analysts considered whether to jump from their windows just after the four o'clock closing bell, I rode the elevator up to the cardiology suite with my father and

Beverly. By the time we rode down again one hour later, a few Wall Street lives had been lost and the value of innumerable stock portfolios stunningly obliterated.

There had also been a prophecy fulfilled: *You have two daughters. One of them will get very sick.*

Dr. Bradley's findings on Black Monday marked the definitive beginning of my life as a sick person on the edge of dying. I would never again know any other kind of life. The stock market, though, recovered and in time reached unprecedented levels of robust trading and widespread prosperity. Some of these profits would come to benefit me directly, helping to pay the massive medical bills that lay ahead.

Madame Clara had been right; she'd seen it all in my father's palm years before: dark and light.

2

ANOTHER HOSPITAL GOWN, THIS TIME A WHITE ONE WITH LITTLE blue pin dots. I left my jeans on and my bra. Dr. Bradley would just have to work around them.

I couldn't tell whether it was something about me that made this seasoned cardiologist appear so uncomfortable, or whether he was just a skittish guy who needed to fidget regardless of the patient lying on his examining table. Even as Dr. Bradley held the stethoscope steady against my chest, he continued to sweep his feet from side to side ever so slightly, in what looked like an abbreviated ballroom dance move. I thought maybe he had to go to the bathroom—with those little nervous shuffles back and forth, back and forth—and then suddenly he came to an abrupt stop. Freeze! He let go of the flat circular end of the stethoscope and left it resting lightly on top of my chest. His hands floated into the air as if someone had just come up behind him and whispered, *Put 'em up real slow.*

I felt my lip begin to curl in an arc of disgust: what was wrong with this guy? A minute ago he couldn't stand still. Now he'd become a statue, an open-mouthed, poorly groomed, stationary block of a man with wild eyes rolled up into his head. This was my new doctor—my cardiologist—the weirdo. I stifled a snicker.

"Well, I think that's enough," he said, the brown centers of his eyes reappearing in their sockets again as he emerged from the fog of listening.

"Why did you do that?"

"What?"

"You just let go of the stethoscope. I've never seen a doctor do that before."

"You haven't been a heart patient before," he said, flashing an imperfect line of yellowish teeth. "Meet me in my office. I'll ask your parents to step in."

"They've never been heart patients either," I said, testing the waters for a sign of humor.

"No matter. You're the patient, right?" Again the yellow smile. "See you inside."

I knew I wasn't going to give this doctor a great big hug. The thought of even having to open my gown for Dr. Bradley's stethoscope again in the future was repulsive. It wasn't like me to be moved to such an extreme level of dislike, but this time I found myself on the lookout for all the things about this particular cardiologist that I could possibly hate. The hostility was new. So was the judgment. I'd never before had any inclination to pick a doctor apart: his physical appearance, his mannerisms, his skill and intelligence as a clinician. But in the wake of being let down so severely by Dr. Clark, I felt free to abandon the kind of worship that had been handed down to me by my father, a man who maintained an almost religious faith in the existence of an all-knowing unassailable higher being known as "the best doctor."

A misdiagnosis from one of these "best doctors" (or a dangerously delayed diagnosis, anyway) had left me with no choice but to break away from my father's belief in medical deities. Dr. Bradley was, after all, just a white-coated guy who'd come recommended by another white-coated guy.

To me, doctors were now just guys.

Sitting with my parents in Dr. Bradley's office just minutes after my examination, it became apparent that this particular medical divinity did not have any easy answers for us. He couldn't explain why my heart was in failure: whether the problem was in the arteries or the muscle, whether it could be treated with medication or not. But he was certain that congestive heart failure in a young person like me was rare and could be quite serious. We would need to determine its root cause as soon as possible in order to avoid "further damage."

Further damage?

Dr. Bradley threw out a few diagnoses that could possibly explain my heart failure. First, my immune system might somehow be implicated and if this were the case, high doses of prednisone, a steroid, could be the solution. In his opinion, this scenario represented the simplest possible cause of my heart problem and was the easiest to resolve. The prednisone would, of course, cause me some unpleasant side effects—things like a thickened neck, a round moon-shaped face, and the possibility of significant weight gain—but if prednisone was all it took to make me better, we'd be lucky.

"I won't take it," I said.

Mistaking my defiance for a lack of understanding, Dr. Bradley slowed his voice down to first-grade-teacher pace and tried again. "I didn't say you had to take it. I'm not even sure if prednisone will help. I only said it was a possibility—the least serious possibility, I believe, at this point."

I had heard him loud and clear the first time; the second go-round only served to heighten my fear. This consultation had become unmanageably scary, deflating my capacity to think clearly and remain calm. The newly bold, keenly critical patient in me began to slip away. In its place came the dreadful sense that I was being forced to take on the concerns and worries of a much, much older person; no part of me—mind, body, or spirit—was equipped to handle heart failure. I began to backpedal, moving away from everything I'd promised myself about being a smarter, more insistent patient this time. My accumulated years began to fall away from me one by one until I landed in the safe haven of a ten-year-old girl—and a bratty one at that.

"I refuse to take a pill that will make me into a fatso with a tree-trunk neck. If it comes to that, you can just forget it. Why don't *you* go take some prednisone?" I said, jutting my chin forward at my new cardiologist, who'd begun clicking the top of his pen in rapid-fire thumb presses.

Beverly reached over and put her hand on my forearm, "Amy, listen to the doctor. He didn't say that you need to take prednisone for sure—"

"I won't take it! I won't!"

Dr. Bradley stopped fidgeting and looked at me in wide-eyed bewilderment from across the desk. I noticed with a wave of renewed revulsion that he'd suddenly become a mouth breather, his tongue resting on his bottom lip just the way it had when he listened to my heart—hands free—a few minutes earlier. He quickly blinked himself back into the present moment and reached for the pen he'd let fall onto his desk. Then, with the sound of my threat still ringing in his ears, Dr. Bradley began to scribble feverishly—line after line—on a fresh piece of paper he'd pulled from my chart. I looked down at the floor in uncomfortable silence, feeling like a bad kid who'd been forced to sit and watch the school principal write a tell-all letter home, only I was a grown woman and the principal had morphed into a cardiologist whose good favor might figure in saving my life.

It was a lapse in behavior that would stay with me forever. The words written in my chart that day would, as it turned out, move along with me into the future as part of my permanent medical record when referrals were made on my behalf among physicians. Nearly every doctor involved with my heart transplant would know that according to the veritable sage Dr. Daniel Bradley—a cardiologist who had made *New York* magazine's elite list of Best Doctors—I was a patient who had some issues. For one, I was emotionally fragile. Also, there was a chance I might be noncompliant, a characterization apt to make doctors recoil.

Dr. Bradley jerked his head up and out of his writing. All of a sudden he had an announcement to make—in a bright, newly energized chirp. "Okay, here's the deal. I won't start you on any prednisone right now. How's that, okay? But I need to put you in the hospital for some tests—just two of them, fairly routine stuff. Once I have the results, we can talk about whether you need steroids or not."

I agreed with a slow nod, content to have scored at least a temporary victory on the prednisone front.

"So we're all set then? Fine. My assistant will make arrangements for your hospital stay," he said, rushing to conclude our meeting. He pushed himself out of his chair and began to stand up. I couldn't help but curl my lip at him one last time, his body language stood in such obvious contradiction to his final words. "Any questions?"

About two dozen of them, yes.

I shook my head no. My parents said thank you. They'd already heard the best-case scenario—the prednisone possibility—and it was their tacit intention to escape Dr. Bradley's office without our having to hear anything worse.

I just wanted to get the hell out of there.

In the elevator, my father looked straight ahead at the closed doors for the whole ride down. When we reached the lobby, he swung his hands around in front of him in a single clap. "Good, then everything is in order," he said. "The man is on it."

This meant Dr. Bradley: medical god.

I waved good-bye to my parents and slipped inside a telephone booth just off the lobby. It was an old-style cubicle with inlaid wood and a glass-paned door that closed tight with a thump that felt like privacy. Alone at last (I'd passed on my father's offer for a ride downtown), I dropped onto the red leather seat and fumbled for enough change to make the call to Philadelphia. My fingers couldn't dial fast enough. The tight space between me and the glass door was palpable; the air had become like wet cement, impossible to take in without opening my mouth as wide as I possibly could and fighting for it. Each successive breath became more of a struggle, until finally I was in an all-out gasp. I'd already loaded the proper change into the pay phone, and now all I had to do was wait a few seconds until the call went through. At once, I became unnaturally aware of my heartbeat. The pounding in my chest was now a magnet, pulling my focus inward and opening my mind to the thought that I might not live beyond this telephone call; my sick heart might not be able to withstand the acute panic coursing through my bloodstream. I became afraid that if I didn't calm the pounding immediately, something terrible might happen.

Maybe this dark wooden phone booth would be my coffin!

Think of something pleasant. Sing. Whistle. Count backwards. Breathe.

Scott answered on the first ring.

"Please come—it's bad," I said. It was all I could manage.

"Oh, my girl. . . ."

He would be on the next train to New York.

Scott and I had known each other only four months by then, but he dropped everything to be by my side. There was not even a question that he would come. Within minutes of hanging up the phone, Scott was on his way, out the door of his apartment, barely stopping to stuff some clean underwear and a toothbrush into his knapsack. He could think of nothing else but his Amy; he had to go to her right now—no matter what.

It was something out of a movie. I'd always remember my Philadelphia phone call that way, as part of a film, with sad music in the background and dramatic low lighting. Like *Love Story*, where a beautiful young coed coughs a few times, appears a little drawn around the eyes, and then turns out to have cancer. The young beauty dies, of course, and her boyfriend is beyond heartbroken because, really, he is not just a boyfriend: he is the man whom destiny has chosen to marry this wonderful girl and be with her forever. He is her love, the truest love there could ever be.

For me, this man would be Scott.

Scott and I met for the first time at a welcoming breakfast buffet in the conference room of a large New York City law firm. We'd both landed summer jobs as law associates, and neither one of us looked quite ourselves on our first day, having ditched our jeans for suits. I wore a serious skirt and matching suit jacket with a camisole underneath; Scott wore gray flannel, his pants several inches too long, pooling on the floor around his loafers. His walk had an unassuming, shuffling quality that was all-out cute as he made his way over to introduce himself. His wide smile arrived steps before his hidden feet did, and it caught me up.

Scott would recount this day many times in the years that followed. He'd scoop me up in his arms for no apparent reason and remind me, with love in his eyes so clearly undiluted by the passage of time, that he knew from the moment he'd seen me snag those two fist-size blueberry muffins (not just one but two, he'd recall) that I was going to be his girl. I'd offered him the second muffin once we began talking, and he ate it, even though he was neither a breakfast eater nor a big fan of blueberries. "It was a price I was willing to pay," he'd say, toying with me in dramatic voice. "I would eat blueberries only for you, my love. You were a vision that morning, in your beige suit with the black lines and that little tank-top thing—"

"It was a camisole." I'd always correct him on this point, playfully, just to break the stride of compliments even as I reveled in them.

I never threw that suit away. It would forever serve to remind me of my silly boyfriend, Scott—how I laughed at him the night he'd told me over and over as he lay on the bathroom floor after too many tequila shots at a law firm bash, "I love you! I love you! I love you!" and then threw up.

"You're drunk," I remembered saying to him, though I also remembered smiling ear to ear. I loved him back and then some.

It all began at that first breakfast; we stood way off in the corner by ourselves. In the first few minutes of chatter, we realized that we'd gone to the same high school, only Scott graduated two years ahead of me, in Jodie's class. His face seemed vaguely familiar at first and then brought to mind a picture from my sister's senior yearbook, which I had pored over to the point of near memorization back when I was a sophomore in search of cute upperclassmen. The photograph was of Scott in blue jean overalls and a plaid flannel shirt. His girlfriend sat square on his lap, her carton of chocolate milk open on the table in front of her. They looked only at each other, captivated. Scott gazed hard into her eyes, clenching his teeth into the kind of smile that comes when something is so damn adorable you can hardly stand it.

It was because of this yearbook photo that one of the first emotions I would connect with Scott would be jealousy, even though his high school girlfriend had long become just a memory for him. To see someone adore another person that way—with teeth—made me want some for myself. One snapshot had told me all I needed to know about the good-looking law associate standing beside me with a blueberry muffin in his hand: he was a man capable of a kind of love I had never known.

On the night before my hospitalization, Scott stayed with me in my father's apartment, which was much closer to New York Hospital than my law dorm downtown. Reluctantly, we sacrificed our privacy for convenience's sake. We would have only this one night together; Scott would spend the next three at my father's without me.

We slept in the old bedroom where I'd spent so many weekends as a child and then as a teenager. The young-girl touches were still intact. My father made it clear to both of us that this coed sleeping arrangement in my room was a special circumstance made possible only by Dr. Bradley's orders that I not exert myself. Scott and I said we understood and then raced down the hall, holding back our laughter until we'd closed the door behind us. We tossed the stuffed animals off the small white bed and laughed into the laced-trimmed pillowcases.

This was the night I first taught myself how to breathe Scott in. It was a practice that would continue on many of our nights together, though he never knew it—or, if he did, he never mentioned it to me. Never once would he ever turn over and say, "Hey, what are you doing?" This was fortunate, because I couldn't possibly explain myself, not in a meaningful way. To breathe Scott in would mean taking from him something that he wouldn't understand exactly how to give, even if he tried.

I'd start by pulling off my T-shirt and drawstring pajama pants (Scott would already be naked, as always in bed), and then I'd turn on my side and align my body point by point with his: feet, knees, pelvis, abdomen, chest, chin, and forehead. Next, I'd open both my hands and spread my fingers out as far as they'd go. This left me with the broadest possible surface area on my palms. With my hands splayed out this way, I'd then place them on Scott's body, usually on the sides of his thighs or hips. Once I had my palms pressed flat against him, I'd relax my fingers and begin to breathe him—in, only. Never out.

I inhaled Scott through my hands.

Sometimes it was his inherent goodness that I'd breathe in, especially on days when I felt angry or mean. But on this night—the long sleepless night before my first hospital admission—I put my open palms against Scott's body and breathed in his health. I had lost mine so suddenly; I knew he would be happy to share.

3

I ARRIVED AT NEW YORK HOSPITAL WITH A LARGE TEDDY BEAR IN tow. My friend Jill bought him for me, having gone straight to FAO Schwarz the moment she heard I would be hospitalized for a series of heart tests. At first I thought her gift silly. But as the weekend passed and my admission date drew nearer, I began to appreciate the bear's hidden assets: a good-sized huggable plumpness—thirty-six inches long with a paunch—touchable, soft, teddy fur; beanbag hands and feet for squishing repeatedly when nervous tension set in. It would turn out that Jill had given me the best present after all, one that fit my needs perfectly. This should not have come as a surprise; Jill and I had been the best of friends since second grade, and almost no one knew me as well as she did.

Today, feeling not at all embarrassed by my very apparent stuffed toy, I sat with Teddy positioned next to me, atop my suitcase, while a hospital admissions person took me through some administrative paces.

"Can you hold out your left hand," she said.

This was not a question.

A green plastic bracelet made its way around my wrist without my assistance. The band displayed my name in small letters next to a more prominent hospital ID number. The admissions person secured the end of it with some kind of adhesive maneuver and finished with a firm press that made me feel anxious—had I just agreed to something important without knowing what it was? My first instinct was to pull at the bracelet with my right hand and check to see if I could stretch the plastic. Maybe take it off later when I was alone in my room.

"Wouldn't do that if I was you," she said. "You don't want to wind up lying in a hallway somewhere without it. No one will know who you are."

"I'll know who I am."

Apparently, I'd made a joke. The hospital admissions person chuckled deep down to her belly. "You have a sense of humor; that's great." She tugged at my bracelet one last time to make sure it was secure. "Oh, look, here comes your ride."

A wheelchair had arrived to take me to my room. My father and Beverly looked away as it came to a stop by the door. "This can't be for me," I said.

But of course it was. Now that I'd finished answering all the admissions questions and had been made an official patient by means of a green plastic band, it was time to go up to the heart floor and begin my hospitalization in earnest. And what better way for someone with congestive heart failure to do this but in a wheelchair?

So far everything about my hospital admission felt like it had been meant for someone else. I had been asked questions that seemed to have no relevance whatsoever to my life, like whether or not I used a cane, wore dentures, or was able to dress myself without assistance. No part of the routine admissions inquiry asked how many times a day I walked up and down the spiral staircase in the law school building, whether I was able to study into the late hours without loss of energy or focus, or what kind of birth control I used—all questions that would have been more appropriate. On the occasion of my first hospital admission, it seemed that the only thing that really mattered about me was that I was a very sick person.

Very sick people, I would soon realize, were expected to ride in hospital wheelchairs without complaint. They had to wear bracelets that would identify them by number rather than name. They were given hospital gowns to wear at all times; embarrassingly revealing round-the-clock pajamas with a long slit up the back that served to remind the wearer that the safest, most dignified place for them to stay was in bed. Very sick hospital patients were expected to put aside all aspects of themselves that were unrelated to their illness. Feelings, thoughts, and fears were just a sorry waste of everyone's time and only served to interfere with a smooth nonconfrontational inpatient experience.

It would not matter to any nurse or doctor during my hospital stay that I was at least forty years too young for serious heart disease. Nor would anyone care to know that the thought of having a sick heart scared me beyond endurance. First-time patients like me were supposed to let go of their healthy selves like sand through the fingers. The loss had to be accepted right away—with a bullet between the teeth, if necessary—and quietly. Passive acceptance was the key to success as a hospital patient: shut up and take it.

I was expected to take an IV into my vein right away, even though the diagnostic testing would not begin until the next morning. Just minutes after I reached my hospital room (on foot, with a large teddy bear taking my place in the wheelchair), a woman came in with a wicker basket stuffed full with needles and vials. She let me know in a singsong voice that she'd be putting in my IV now.

"No one said I'd need an IV today."

"All patients in hospital get IV," she said.

"Not this one."

The cheerful basket woman, who'd now identified herself as the IV and blood-drawing technician, made a clucking sound with her tongue. She removed the load of ammunition from the crook of her arm and placed it at the end of my bed. I hadn't yet changed into a hospital gown, nor had I gotten under the covers; it was early afternoon, and I'd refused to cooperate with an order that would have me wear a piece of backless cloth and spend the next few hours in it, staring up at my father, Beverly, and Scott from a hospital bed.

I'd already told the nurse that I wasn't ready for sleep—or for hospital nightwear, for that matter—at two-thirty in the afternoon. She had been just about to respond through pursed lips when the wicker basket lady came swinging through my door.

"I think your family had better wait outside until we're done here, okay, Mommy, Daddy?" The IV tech sent my parents and Scott out of the room with a sharp upward thrust of her chin. Scott widened his eyes at me as he walked out. He could not believe that I would be this difficult.

My opponent and I were left to face off over the wicker basket, but we were not alone in the room. The floor nurse remained with us, her arms crossed over her chest as if waiting to see what this uncooperative snot-ass patient was going to do now.

It was only five minutes into my hospital stay, and already I'd earned myself a bad reputation.

"If you don't let me do this, I'll have to get some help down the hall. You don't want to be held down, do you?" Apparently, since my family had left the room, it was now all right for the basket woman to threaten me.

"Fuck you," I said.

The IV tech had heard enough. She scooped her arm through the curve of the basket, exhaled loudly, and flew out of my room in quick, small steps. Suddenly I realized that my parents had left the door open on their way out and my "Fuck you" could have reached their ears—or, worse, Scott's. I felt a pang of embarrassment, but not one strong enough to change my mind.

Help arrived from down the hall. Two more nurses appeared at my door, one with tree-trunk arms and the other with a scowl that meant unpleasant business. The IV tech crept by them, slipping back into my room to finish the job. She was supposed to be the expert at putting patients at ease—at least the ones who weren't crazy. The insertion of this IV would be a test only of my sanity, then, not of her skill. She sat down on my bed and asked if I would please sit beside her—just for a minute. This basket, she said sweetly, had been to every single room on this floor, and three other floors as well, day after day, for five years, if I could believe it. These little tiny needles—she pulled out a few wrapped samples to show me—were just a regular everyday part of being in the hospital. Smile, smile. Nothing unusual about them at all. IVs were for every patient. And really the needle wasn't that bad.

Seeing as I still hadn't been won over, the scowl-face sentry nurse stationed by the door tried to shame me with a throaty reminder that I was "twenty-four years old for heaven's sake" and "even the children don't act like this."

The basket lady agreed. She gave up on the sweet talk and barked at me instead. "Give me your arm!"

A scream came up from a dark wretched place inside me that I didn't know existed. I'd never heard anything like it come out of me before. The piercing sound launched my body out the door, past the tree-trunk arms and disapproving faces, and down the long hallway in one sustained high-pitch shriek: "No-o-o-o-o!" A hostile audience watched from my room back at the other end of the hall. A couple of patients' heads peeped out of doorways to see what the screaming was all about.

Oh, that's just Dr. Bradley's patient. *Fragile,* the chart said.

Scott came to retrieve me by the patients' lounge. I heard his sneakers, slow and steady, squeaking their way toward me on the hallway tiles. The pace of his step gave me a good twenty seconds to begin feeling awfully ashamed of myself. By the time he reached me I was sobbing, ready to throw myself at his feet and beg to be forgiven for what he'd just witnessed. He opened his arms to me and I fell into them like a rag doll, embarrassment wedged uncomfortably between us. He took my hand and we walked back to my room together, past the nurses, who'd already returned to their more routine duties, and past my parents, who looked down at their feet. Scott asked if he could have a minute alone with me and shut the door.

I sat on the edge of the bed. Scott paced in front of me and then stopped. "I know you're upset about this hospitalization, but you can't act like this, you just can't," he said, more insistent than I'd ever before heard him. "The people in this hospital—doctors, nurses, technicians—they're all here to help you. You must know that, right?"

I wasn't so sure, but I knew my behavior had to change—right away.

Scott expected more from me than I had given today; I'd failed him by treating people badly. Part of his vast capacity for love, I knew then for sure, was a deep consideration and respect for the feelings of others. The well-meaning hospital staff was foremost in his mind. They deserved only appreciation and cooperation, not my wrath, he said. Scott taught me many things about kindness on that first day in the hospital.

In the days and years to come, I would teach him some things as well—about unrelenting illness and what it can do to the gentle manners of those afflicted by it. But for now I would only say that I was truly sorry for my behavior. I chose not to tell him just how terrified I'd been—how I felt almost certain that I was going to die from this heart thing, whatever it was. My scream down the hallway had not been the cry of a grown-up baby; it was the chilling sound of a young woman coming smack up against the thought of her death.

Scott sat alongside me while the IV nurse slid a needle into my forearm. Afterward he set out to walk the ten blocks to my father's apartment alone. Back in my childhood room, under the lace-edged comforter and surrounded by my stuffed animals, Scott began to cry. He told me later that he had cried like this every night for the remainder of my hospital stay.

4

A HEART BIOPSY IS A KIND OF TORTURE THAT NO PERSON SHOULD have to endure—not even once. It entails the removal of heart tissue from a patient who, most often, is not offered any sedation. A bit of local anesthetic is the most a heart biopsy patient can hope for—injected into the neck. This painkiller's efficacy is sorely limited.

Neither heart nor patient tends to react to the biopsy procedure very well. There is something profoundly unnatural, if not entirely counterintuitive, about snipping off vital tissue from a pulsing life-giving organ. Even the healthiest of hearts is apt to buck and sputter in revolt during biopsy, breaking into arrhythmic beats as the pincer-grip end of the catheter moves in for the taking. Patients may cry out when they feel pieces of their hearts being snatched from them this way. They are likely to perceive the maneuver as a nasty yank (not the little tug that biopsy doctors promise), and the sensation is often more than just pain; heart biopsy can be experienced as an act of cruelty.

I had my first biopsy at New York Hospital as part of the "fairly routine" tests scheduled for me by Dr. Bradley. Even as my stretcher rolled into the exam room, I did not have a clear idea of what a biopsy entailed. I knew only that I was supposed to be in good hands (Dr. Bradley had selected my biopsy doctor personally) and that the results of the exam would provide important information about my heart failure. No one told me that the medical term *biopsy* meant excision of living tissue—heart tissue, in my case—and I didn't think to ask. Why would I expect a routine exam to include plucking out pieces of my heart? When I lay down on the stretcher, there was no reason for me to fear the worst; I didn't even know what the worst could possibly be. But I emerged from the exam room ninety minutes later with enough unwanted knowledge, experience, and trauma to fill my head with a dozen bloodcurdling nightmares.

When Dr. Bradley came to see me in my hospital room later that day, I told him the exam had been beyond awful. He said he was sorry to hear it and offered up as consolation some words to the effect of "Well, at least it's behind you now." He then sought to reduce the chance of any emotional aftershocks by suggesting that my first heart biopsy would also be my last.

In fact, Dr. Bradley turned out to be wrong.

Proof of this would come down to a count that began on this biopsy day and continued for years to come. Over time, I added them up and found that I'd white-knuckled my way through nearly sixty-five heart biopsies. It had been promised to me early on by overly optimistic cardiologists that researchers would soon come up with a better way than biopsy to gather vital diagnostic information. But almost two decades later I still found myself lying on the familiar narrow table in the biopsy suite at periodic intervals, with a sterile plug stuck in my neck and a catheter threaded through it, hearing the same hollow promise that medical science was coming close—no, really close this time—to an alternative. Meanwhile, I would have to abide doctors snipping away at my life source because biopsy was the one and only test that could determine—definitively—my heart's health. Regularly scheduled biopsies became a necessary evil for my survival; every so often one of the doctors would remind me—as I lay on the exam table—that even though biopsy was an admittedly "uncomfortable" procedure, it was a small price to pay for being alive, wasn't it?

I wondered whether the person who first put forth that paper-thin rationalization had ever lain down for a biopsy—let alone for more than sixty of them. I asked Dr. Waller about it once, years after my first heart biopsy at New York Hospital. He'd just pulled a long catheter from my neck for the tenth time in five minutes and emptied a tiny slice of my heart muscle onto a microscope slide. I knew all too well that he would need to retrieve four usable pieces in order to complete the biopsy, but so far he'd only been able to produce one. Ten separate yanks at my heart had yielded mostly pitiful bits of scar tissue: these were the unusable samples that turned up whenever the catheter snipped at a spot in the heart where a biopsy had already been taken at some time in the past. All the years of snips and rips had turned my heart into a minefield of fibrous scarring and turned Dr. Waller's job into a fishing expedition to locate and reel in four rare pieces of live tissue. Sometimes it would take him thirty tries to do it.

"Any doctor you know ever gone through this—had a heart biopsy himself?" I asked, the sound of my voice vibrating through the antiseptic plastic draping that lay over my face.

"Nope."

"Don't you think it would be a good idea if one of you guys did, just so you'd know what it's like?"

"No, I do not. Especially not me, thank you. Now lie still, please. I'm going in again. No talking." I felt the end of the catheter sharp against my skin as it entered my neck for the eleventh time.

"Uh-oh, sorry," he said. "Didn't get anything that time either." Dr. Waller had just pulled out another useless blank.

"Tell me, dear doctor, how many times a day do you say *I'm sorry?*" After so many years of biopsies together, Dr. Waller and I had gotten used to ribbing each other this way.

"Before or after I go home to my wife?"

Boy, he was quick! And he got me again—managed to extract a laugh right in the middle of a heart biopsy that was going quite badly for both of us. He waited for the wave of chuckles to circulate among the eavesdropping nurses and technicians in the room and then plunged the catheter into my neck for another try.

All gaiety was on hold once again. I shut my eyes tight and bit down as hard as I could, contorting my face muscles like a weightlifter struggling his way into a monstrous thrust overhead.

The ordeal of the heart biopsies never lessened over time. There was the physical pain involved, of course; no one likes to have a plug stuffed into her neck like a cork, not even if you were lucky enough to have two injections of local numbing medicine. But worse than the needle stings and the knife slice in my neck, which often turned my skin black-and-blue overnight, was the unnerving sensation of my heart bouncing wildly in response to the catheter invading its sacred space. It scared me. When my heart bumped around this way, it would show up on the EKG screen as a string of abnormal beats—arrhythmias—which would then prompt the biopsy nurse to call out "V!" Dr. Waller would be glad to hear it, because V meant ventricle, and once it was determined that the errant heartbeats were originating from the ventricle, he could be sure the catheter had made its way to prime biopsy territory and the plucking could begin.

During my first-ever heart biopsy at New York Hospital, the Vs felt like nothing at all; I barely noticed them. Dr. Bradley hadn't told me that part of my diagnostic testing might involve the induction of some irregular heartbeats, so I was not watching out for strange sensations in my chest. And even if I were to feel some odd pulsations weaving in and out of my normal heartbeat, I would have reacted completely without alarm; I didn't know that heartbeats could themselves be dangerous—even lethal. All I knew (or thought I knew) was that heart attacks were the cardiac events to be feared, and that these happened to old people—usually overweight ones who smoked and ate too much fatty meat. I also thought, wrongly, that cardiac trouble always came in the form of a sudden crushing pain in the chest. On TV shows and in the movies, a heart attack victim would collapse to the floor, a gasping helpless soul just barely able to mumble his last words: *The pain, oh, the terrible pain!* But, of course, that was just the storybook version of death by heart attack; it wasn't how things really happened.

In time, I would learn that cardiac death can come without any chest discomfort at all. It can start as a vague feeling of *I'm not right,* followed by a more certain feeling that something is awfully wrong, and then end in a quick, quiet, painless collapse. There was a lot more for me to fear than just prednisone, clogged arteries, and chest pain after all.

When Dr. Bradley told me that the results of one of the diagnostic tests he'd ordered—the angiogram—had shown that my arteries were completely normal, with no blockages or narrowing, I became almost giddy with relief. Whatever might be wrong with my heart, I now believed, it was not going to land me face down on the carpet, clutching my chest. No matter how sick I was, my death wouldn't hit me suddenly in the middle of a quiet conversation or on a city bus.

My arteries were too healthy for that.

But it did bother me that Dr. Bradley didn't seem as relieved as I was by the good news of my angiogram. He said he'd expected the results to come out fine all along, and he had only ordered the test to confirm his earliest suspicions: that the cause of my congestive heart failure had nothing to do with my arteries. Dr. Bradley still awaited the result of the biopsy because he believed that the tissue samples would tell him things he didn't already know.

Then, just twenty-four hours after my first heart biopsy, Dr. Bradley stood at the foot of my hospital bed and set me straight. "The tissue samples indicate that you have—or you had, at some time—a virus in your heart. There is some scarring. It seems to suggest that the damage may be on the mend, but—"

"Will I have to take prednisone?" I interrupted, with a question that was, at least for me, burning and quite obvious. To Dr. Bradley, it was a dumbfounding non sequitur. He looked into my eyes for the first time since entering my hospital room, then opened his mouth yawn-wide and let his tongue hang a little, just like he'd done when my words had caught him off guard a few days earlier in his office. It was an ugly off-putting pose that Dr. Bradley would fall into from time to time in my presence, when an uncomfortable mixture of nonlinear thought and creeping disdain welled up in him.

My question had brought him back into this pose today. "What? prednisone? Oh, that again. No. No prednisone."

Only his last two words had found their way to my ears. I couldn't imagine hearing any better news.

"But you will have to take some other medications—not any of them steroids; don't worry. They're cardiac medications that will take some stress off your heart function. Your heart needs to rest and recover . . . and repair itself, I hope."

There were clues in his words, but I chose to miss them. Everything that was said would remain unexamined because Dr. Bradley and I were alone in the room. No one was there to comb through his words with me so the truth could be extracted: that Dr. Bradley was not very sure of anything just yet—neither the progression of the virus in my heart nor its prognosis. The heart biopsy had not provided us with an answer; it had only made a few suggestions.

"So I had some kind of virus in my heart for some reason, and now my heart is getting better?"

"It looks that way."

"Right. When can I go home?"

"I'd like to keep you here for a couple more days while you get started on a few different medicines. I want to see how you do on them before you leave."

By the end of our conversation, I had pieced together a patchwork story of my test results that served me sufficiently well.

Later that day, I relayed to my parents and Scott what I'd heard Dr. Bradley say. I never knew whether any of them then went on to have a separate conversation with him as well. If they did, they never told me about it and never attempted to realign my wishful thinking with a more accurate description of the test results. To them, my diagnosis was very much a wait-and-see kind of situation anyway, so there would be no hurry to correct my take on it. If my murky understanding of the facts had allowed me to keep my head in a positive cloud as time passed, all the better. The important thing was to keep me moving forward: up and out of the hospital, back to law school, and on with my life. This would require everyone around me to shut their eyes for the time being.

I left the hospital two days after receiving this diagnosis from Dr. Bradley. At the time of my discharge, I was deemed sufficiently acclimated to all the heart medications that were running through my bloodstream for the first time. But I hardly felt used to taking them; I'd never needed to take any pill on a daily basis before, and now I had to swallow several—all cardiac related and none of them optional. I would have to be sure to take every pill every day because, I was told, each one of them was vital to my recovery.

There, I'd heard it again: that dulcet word *recovery*.

My heart was going to get better, all better. It was just a matter of taking some pills, and surely I could do that. I was ready to be a good patient now.

Back in my dorm some weeks later, my suite mate's dog ate some remains of my heart medicine out of the wastebasket under my desk. I must have forgotten to close the door to my room when I left for class in the morning, because when I returned later, the basket lay on its side with all its contents splayed out. Half-chewed tissues and crumpled paper settled into wet, mushy mounds on the floor, a pill bottle ominously among them with its cover nowhere to be found. When I'd tossed the bottle in the trash the night before, it contained shavings of pills that I had made unusable by splitting them in half unsuccessfully (half doses were a necessary prescription for a small-boned lightweight like me). Now my pills were on their way to Dunkin's stomach. Upon discovering this fearsome sight, Dunkin's owner, Valerie, called her vet in a fit of panic. Through tears of hysteria, she begged him to tell her the truth: was her puppy within minutes of a heart attack?

The vet laughed for longer than Valerie appreciated and then asked what drug had been in the basket. What was its function?

This question was mine to answer. I quickly told Valerie the trademark name and my sense that it was supposed to be a *vasodilator,* or something like that. But I admitted that I didn't understand what that term meant exactly; I didn't really know the functions of my own heart medications.

I didn't want to know.

Smart, savvy patients are not born; they are made—sometimes unwillingly. My education would begin with a reluctant lesson in identifying and articulating the side effects of my medications. Before I left the hospital, Dr. Bradley asked me whether the drugs I'd been taking for the previous forty-eight hours had made me feel anything. I didn't realize he was asking specifically about side effects. As far as I knew, most medications (besides prednisone) didn't have any effects other than their intended ones: aspirin eased headaches, antibiotics cured strep throat, and cortisone cream relieved the itch of poison ivy—there wasn't much more to it than that. Medicines were supposed to make people better, and mine were on their way to doing just that. I was on the look out only for sensations related to my impending cure—not for unpleasant or worrisome side effects—and I imagined I felt the earliest indications of improved health even before my discharge from the hospital. The new sensation of heaviness in my arms and the general sluggishness I experienced were actually good signs, I thought, since I'd been told that my medications would allow my heart to rest and recover. It sure felt like the pills were doing a great job. My heart had already begun its restorative relaxation; I could tell. Most of my energy had been sapped in the process, but this could only mean that the medicines were giving my heart the break it needed.

Right?

I told Dr. Bradley that I thought I was feeling better. Over the next few months, I would say the same thing to my law school classmates and to Scott as well. I'd be damned if any part of my body was going to slow me down. My heart may have failed for a while—but *I* would not fail.

In the months after my hospitalization, there would be many opportunities to test this resolve. Once, after rushing through the rain to reach a late-day seminar on time, I arrived in the lobby of the law school building, dropped my umbrella on the floor by the entrance, and lifted my head up into complete blindness. My first instinct was not to give in to whatever was happening to me; rather than focus on my body, I focused my attention on my surroundings. I reached out for the wall and stepped in close to it, feeling embarrassed and not wanting the other students to notice that there was an emergency going on. I bent my head forward and pretended to rummage in my bag for something, but my eyes continued to see only what I could hear. Finally, little streaks of light and color began to flicker in front of me and my sight returned. I ran up the spiral staircase to the first floor and realized for the first time that my heart was dancing madly, stealing the air from my lungs. Again, I shoved my hand deep into my bag and pretended to look for something vitally important. Just as my breath came back to me, I found the all-consuming item I'd been digging for: my pen.

Some years later, after experience had infused me with all kinds of knowledge about sick hearts and the sneaky ways they show themselves, I would look back on my moment of blindness and think about what it might have been: a blood clot, a stroke. I had stood in the lobby of NYU law school and experienced a very quiet, dignified cardiac episode, all the while working hard to appear normal. And then when the episode had passed, I gritted my teeth and forged on; I had a seminar to attend, damn it.

It may have been ignorance that prevented me from putting a name on my symptoms that day, but it was my willpower that swept me up and away from the frightening mystery that stole my sight. No matter how much I had wanted to grab one of my friends in the lobby and share my terror, I would keep my hands—and my worsening illness—to myself. I was convinced it was the better way for me to go; health problems at twenty-four could be such a downer.

I realized from the earliest stages of my illness that the people around me responded better when I stayed strong and kept all the ugly details to myself. The story of my wild run down the hall from the IV nurse—I learned with shame and self-recrimination—did not win me respect and accolades. Smiles did. A positive outlook did. So did a tightly buttoned lip. My school friends loved the illusion I created on our daily walks to the law building. I could read in their faces how pleased they were to see me resume my regular law school life in spite of the diagnosis of congestive heart failure. I liked hearing all those emphatic *You're amazing!* comments and the comparisons that pointed up how seamlessly I'd moved on; more than one of my classmates told me, "If I were you, I would have taken a leave of absence this semester for sure." The thought had never occurred to me.

I fed my friends a whole lot of sunshine as my illness progressed, and they soaked it right up. No one dared question me; I looked great, I acted fine, I handed my papers in on time, and I kept the gory details of heart biopsies, angiograms, and attacks of blindness, weakness, and breathlessness to myself. Pretty soon, everyone forgot about my hospitalization and the diagnosis I'd received there.

It was even Dr. Bradley's impression that I looked well and seemed energetic at my next checkup. My heart didn't sound worse than it had before. But once Dr. Bradley glanced down at the markings on the EKG strip emerging through the end of the machine, he could no longer be fooled by appearances. The up-and-down black lines didn't hold back the truth; they told the story of every scary symptom I'd kept to myself over the previous two months. My heart had grown weaker. The medicines were not helping. The virus in my heart didn't seem to be on the mend after all.

"Let me show you something here." Dr. Bradley took the EKG strip and laid it down on the countertop next to a nearly identical strip from my previous office visit. I slid off the exam table and came over to take a look. "See this line, the way it dips down? Last time you were here, it dipped slightly less. See?" He took a pencil and circled the corresponding line on the earlier EKG. "Just so you know—less dip is better."

I thought the two lines looked pretty much the same, it was my first time studying an EKG up close. Before long I would become a near expert in the interpretation of my EKGs, but for now I had to rely on Dr. Bradley's skills to provide me with an accurate—and honest—reading.

"Of course, EKG machines aren't perfect and the change is small, so I can't be sure of what I'm looking at here," he said. "It might mean absolutely nothing; we'll just have to wait and see. And besides, you have a scan coming up next month, don't you?"

I did. Another diagnostic test—a new and different one that was considered part of my outpatient follow-up—had already been scheduled for me at an upscale private cardiac testing facility outside the hospital. Dr. Bradley assured me that the results of this exam would provide a lot more information than could be provided by an EKG strip. Meanwhile, I shouldn't worry; he'd see me in eight weeks, and we'd put all the pieces together.

But even before I returned to Dr. Bradley's office, the puzzle was solved. A talky technician at the cardiac testing facility prattled his way into revealing the results of my scan—in so many words—even though I hadn't asked. He began chatting me up while inserting my IV (which I allowed him to do without protest) and then continued to engage me while injecting precise doses of radioactive isotopes and tagging substances that would reveal the strength of my heart muscle. After I was fully injected, he laid me down on the exam table, centered some kind of camera over my chest, and left me there while he went off to observe the data collection from another room.

Later, when the test was done, I walked out of the dressing area and found the technician waiting for me in the hall, ready as ever to talk.

"So, uh . . . how are you feeling?" he asked, leaning one shoulder against the wall.

"Good. Fine."

"Really?" He lifted his chin in the air and peered down his nose at me with squinting eyes that could have been either flirty or challenging, depending on how you looked at them

"Yeah. Why?"

"Well, it's just . . . I was thinking. What kinds of things do you do every day?"

"I go to law school. I'm in class for about six hours most days, and then I study a lot. On weekends I take a train to Philadelphia to see my boyfriend." I paused to let the *boyfriend* sink in. "I'm really, really busy."

I was almost sure this guy was trying to pick me up.

"And you're telling me you feel fine?"

"Pretty much, yeah." My answer came slowly and with downcast eyes; only now did I understand where this talky technician had been going with these questions. He'd just seen the results of my scan.

I moved in with the best defense I could muster: "I know things might not look great on paper, but I have to say, the medicines really do help. They make it so my heart doesn't have to pump so hard, you know? And I can go and go all day long. . . ." My words hit the air with an awkward, false ring.

The technician broke into a friendly grin that said he wanted to believe what I'd just told him but didn't. "It's amazing that you feel so well. Those pills must be something else, huh?"

"Must be. 'Cause I feel fine. Lots of energy."

"Well, great. Good for you. It's hard to believe, though, I gotta say. The scan showed some pretty low heart function."

I put aside this troubling statement, figuring I'd get a better answer a few days later at my next appointment. I joined Dr. Bradley at the countertop so that, together, we could compare my latest EKG strip with the previous ones. Even before his guiding pencil hit the page, I had already studied the latest strip unassisted and had a sense of what it revealed: the last two months had been a time of great change. Somehow the little dip had turned into a significant plunge.

Just as dramatically, I had become a much smarter patient. I'd learned how to recognize a bad EKG.

5

THERE WERE FLOWERS WAITING FOR ME AT MY DORM WHEN I RE-turned from the doctor. Roses. A dozen of them peeked out from behind the counter where a security guard sat checking IDs. As I approached the desk, I saw him lean over and grab hold of the clear plastic wrapping that held the latest shipment of Scott's love; it was the sixth or seventh flower delivery I'd received from him since the summer ended.

The best part was always the card: a few words written in the hand of a local florist according to Scott's precise direction. Sometimes there would just be a laugh, like today: *I smell for you. Love, Scott*. Unwrapping the small square envelope, I stepped into the elevator and nearly tripped over the foot of a classmate. My world had narrowed to include only the words written on the white card that I now held in my hand.

"Ha! Funny! Oh, God, I love him!"

Without realizing it, I'd blurted out a cry of unrestrained joy to an elevator full of grumpy law students who weren't the least bit interested. The doors opened at my floor, and I floated through them and down the hall to my room. I had a decision to make: should I throw the flowers out right away or wait a few minutes?

From the first bouquet Scott had sent me several months earlier, I had a problem keeping his flowers in my room. I found that they made me wheeze, a reaction that was new for me, as I'd never had an allergy to flowers before. I forced myself to keep September's roses—the first delivery—on my night table right up until they wilted away, even though I could hear my own raspy breath with each exhalation while falling asleep at night. I tolerated the October flowers in the same way, sacrificing several comfortable nights' sleep for the constant reminder of Scott's love. But by the time November came around, I had been diagnosed and hospitalized with congestive heart failure, and it began to dawn on me that the wheezing might have less to do with flowers than with my heart's struggle to pump when I was lying down. From this point on, Scott's roses became a source of worry for me every time they arrived. To push the wheezing problem out of my mind, I decided to get rid of all flower deliveries as soon as they arrived, just in case they were contributing to my breathing difficulties. It made me sad to do it, and I never told Scott I had to.

But I was hiding more than just my flower problem from him. On weekends, when I would visit Scott in Philadelphia, I'd step off the train full of an energy I didn't have and exuding a positive outlook that would become more and more flimsy as time went on. None of it felt like a lie to me, because it wasn't; every moment I spent with Scott was fueled by the most restorative, healing love. I waited all week to leave my cramped dorm room behind and step into Scott's spacious apartment, jumping into his arms and into the queen-size bed that made Penn a much better home for us than NYU. When the moment came when I would have to climb the steep staircase at 30th Street Station that delivered me into Scott's embrace, I was infused with the healthy stamina of the twenty-four-year-old woman I wished I could be. Up those stairs I'd run, sometimes two at a time; halfway there, I'd lift my head and see Scott waiting at the top for me, the white sun shining through the giant windows behind him. His smile was enough to cure me right then and there—at least for as long as it would take to reach him. My

Scotty: he was there for me again, just as he was every Friday afternoon. And I felt fine—really fine—the moment we finally kissed at the stairway's end. Our weekend had begun.

By midday on Saturday, though, the usual heart symptoms would settle in and I'd have to take whatever strength I could from him and hope it would be enough to get me through the weekend without having to give my secret away. One weekend was particularly difficult because Scott had decided that a little Philadelphia tourism—the Liberty Bell—might be fun. We parked our car only a few blocks away from the site, but the walk felt like an uphill trek. Scott put his arm around my shoulders, and the added weight was too much. I was sinking under the heaviness of his ski jacket—as if he'd stuffed sandbags into the sleeves and was playing a trick on me to see how far I could go without falling over. I was just about to tell him to please take his arm away, but then my will overruled me; I was going to finish this walk with Scott's arm wherever he chose to put it, even if I had to crawl on my knees. I set my sights on the bell two blocks ahead in the distance, put my head down into the wind, and began to count my steps forward in a silent, desperate effort to distract my thoughts from my exhausted body, which begged for rest: one . . . two . . . three. . . . Then the tears began to fall. I didn't bother to wipe them away. If Scott asked me about them, I'd just blame it on the stinging March wind. I was courageous and ridiculous—a stubborn young woman determined to overrule her collapsing body. But I was forced to face the truth about my worsening heart condition just days after denying it at the foot of the Liberty Bell: an even lower-dipping EKG showed up at my next doctor's appointment.

Dr. Bradley suggested that I might want to consult a specialist in the field of cardiomyopathy, which was the new name he'd assigned to my illness in light of the latest test results. Cardiomyopathy meant heart muscle damage. We already knew my heart muscle had been damaged, presumably by a virus. But the progression of increasing damage baffled Dr. Bradley; he had been under the impression that the virus was on the mend, not still on the attack. He wasn't really suggesting that I see another doctor; he was telling me I had to do it, because at this point he wasn't sure he could make sense of my illness. A doctor who is a specialist in his field does not often send a patient to another specialist in the same field. Dr. Bradley may have been the best cardiologist in New York City, but there was an excellent doctor at Boston's Massachusetts General Hospital who was willing to see me right away—at the end of this week, if I could make it.

Friday morning I flew to Boston with my father and Beverly.

I thought by now that I was an old pro at lying down for cardiac diagnostic tests, and in many ways, I was—except one: I had never lain down for an exam stone-cold scared of the result. On my back in a dark room at Mass General, I shivered as the technician rolled a sonogram wand back and forth over my left breast, searching for the best view of my heartbeat. I looked over at the black-and-white screen beside my head and saw what looked like a pulsing walnut. It was my heart, I knew, and as far as I could tell it was pumping away without any starts and stops. The technician leaned forward and turned a knob on the screen that must have been volume, because all of a sudden I could hear a whooshing sound, like the inside of an amplified seashell. The noise frightened me, and I shifted my eyes over to the technician for reassurance. She told me it was the sound of my heart; she was going to record sounds from all four chambers along with some pictures and measurements of blood flow. I should just lie back and relax.

Then the test began in earnest. Conversation gave way to silence, and I began to worry again. The technician seemed calm at first, almost indifferent as she moved the wand over the same small section of my chest again and again. Then she changed the angle of her hand, pushed the wand into a spot on my breastbone just left of center, and came to an abrupt stop.

"Huh." The technician tapped a computer key twice. "Huh," she said again, staring with intense interest at the now-paused image on her screen.

And then she was up. "Stay right there, okay? I'll only be a minute."

She already had one foot out the door when I jolted upright, bare-chested, into a sitting position and asked, "Is everything all right?"

"Sure. I could just use another pair of eyes, that's all."

Then she was gone; I'd missed my chance to grab the back of her white coat and plead for an encouraging word. I spent the next ten minutes alone, half naked in a dark exam room, staring with untrained eyes at a frozen computer image. Something in that image had been worthy of a mad dash down the hall.

When the technician returned, she brought back with her not one but eight pairs of eyes: seven awkward young doctors and their gray-haired leader, a professor who couldn't have been more delighted to see me.

"Oh, hello! These are cardiology residents here with me today, and we would be most grateful if you would let us take a peek at your echocardiogram. We do this sort of thing all the time. We're a teaching hospital, you see."

The technician moved aside and allowed the professor to take over her seat and her wand. He dropped down into the chair and began to retrace the area over my heart at double speed, darting from side to side in jerky motions and at odd angles until he hit the same spot that had sent the technician running from my room. Seven white coats moved in around the exam table and nodded in eager agreement with the professor's commentary. "Here it is, folks. See this? And that? You're not going to get to see that very often, so take a close look now, while you can. Most interesting, no?"

Oh, yes. A hum of excitement came up from the young doctor crowd. They'd never seen anything like it. My heart was quite a show. The professor nearly applauded.

One freeze-frame image had been more than enough to satisfy his teaching requirements for the day. "Thanks so much. Really, thank you." He was buoyant, smiling as he gave my hand a delighted squeeze. "We'll be on our way now. Have a nice day." I tried to read the faces of the residents as they filed out of the room, but none of them would lift their eyes to meet my gaze. These young doctors were, I noticed, right around the same age as I was. I'd given them a bit of a fright today—along with a unique learning opportunity.

I was a scary story, no doubt. My illness had made me into one of those people who serves as the protagonist in the kind of thank-god-it's-not-me tale that will run through entire communities and even through young doctors' minds.

Looking at my face in the mirror on the exam room wall, I saw for the first time the reflection of a very unlucky girl. I wiped my tears and joined my parents in the waiting room. Within minutes, my name was called, and we walked together down the hospital corridor to the specialist's office. He greeted us unceremoniously.

He told us that Dr. Bradley had sent to him all my test results and EKGs and that these, along with the preliminary findings on my echocardiogram, led him to believe that it wasn't time to put me on the heart-transplant waiting list just yet.

"We could try to put you on the list now, but it would be a bit of a stretch. We really don't know which way things will go for you. The next six months will tell. Your heart will either get better, or it will get worse," he said.

Heart transplant? What was a heart transplant?

"Dr. Bradley never said anything about a heart transplant," I said.

"He didn't? Well, I'm only saying that I wouldn't put you on the list yet. I think he and I are in agreement."

I searched my parents' faces, but they looked as shocked as I was.

The specialist continued. "For now, you should stay on your current medicines. They might help you. But I can say with near certainty that your heart muscle is sufficiently damaged to prevent you from playing sports—now and in the future—though I don't know how important that is to you. Also, you will not be able to carry a child; your heart muscle will never recover enough to do that, I'm sure. Other than those two prohibitions, we'll have to wait and see."

"But my heart could be well in six months, right?"

"Maybe, but not well enough for sports or pregnancy."

"How can that be—?" I choked on my words and could not go on. The tears had arrived in full force. Beverly moved in, taking her best shot at optimism.

"Doctor, tell me, will she be able to play golf?" she asked.

"I suppose so."

"See, Amy, this is good! You *can* do sports—one of them, at least." She already knew that I didn't consider golf to be a sport at all. In three sentences, this doctor had just erased tennis, jogging, hiking, skiing, and motherhood from my life, and Beverly was trying to appease me with golf as a replacement. I squinted my eyes at her and let go of my good manners and self-control like a belligerent teenager.

"Golf is for old people! I hate golf and I am never ever going to play it."

"Oh, don't be silly," Beverly said. "Lots of young people play golf. At our club, some of the best players are people your age. It's really a terrific sport. You'll see! I bet Scott would like it too! There are so many beautiful places to travel for golf, like Scotland and—"

"That's enough, Beverly." My father interrupted her. "Amy is a big girl. It doesn't matter whether she plays golf or not. What she does with her life is up to her. Now, let's go. We're done here, aren't we?"

The doctor said we were and told me to make an appointment to see him in six months. My father hurried out the door in a huff, leaving me and Beverly to wonder at his sudden burst of anger. We caught up with him at the elevator and knew from his expression that he wanted silence.

There was a taxi waiting outside that would take us to Logan, where my father and Beverly would catch a plane to New York and I would board one for Philadelphia. It was eerily silent in the backseat; Beverly sat in the middle. The tears that had started flowing during the consultation had now turned into an all-out sob that forced my upper body to shudder. I began calling out fragments of despair: *Permanently damaged! Sick heart forever! Never play tennis again! Like an old woman!*

Beverly lifted her arm up behind my neck and let me cry against her shoulder, but this kindness only brought me closer to the sadness I'd been holding in since being forced to play the starring role in the echocardiogram show that day. I began to wail like a teething infant, struggling to get a sentence out between the sobs that punctuated every effort to breathe. "I will never be a mother!"

"That's it!" my father said. The taxi had stopped at a light. He grabbed the car door handle, lifted it in a dramatic motion, and shouted into the air without turning his head in my direction: "I don't have to take this! Come on, Beverly, let's get out of here!"

He flung the door open, jumped out into the middle of the busy street, and waited for Beverly to follow. She slid across the backseat toward the door, shrugged her shoulders at me, and got out after him. The door slammed shut and the taxi continued to the airport with me alone in the backseat.

6

I SAT IN THE THIRD ROW OF A SMALL LECTURE HALL AND CAME AS close as I ever would to praying. All I wanted was for my body to be quiet. The professor had made his way through more than half of the Criminal Procedure lesson for the day, and I didn't think I could hold on much longer. My heart had been Acting Up—a label I'd given to an erratic fluttering in my chest that had become more frequent lately, sending strong, undeniably clear messages that it was on a much shorter time schedule than any doctor had predicted. Erratic heartbeats tugged at my awareness now, right in the middle of an upper-level Crim Pro class that demanded full attention. It was taught by a five foot tall professor who'd earned himself the nickname Little Napoleon for his success in obliterating the egos of brave young men in the first two rows of seats and for making women cry wherever they chose to sit—or hide—in the classroom.

I begged fate not to let the professor find me today. I knew that the odds were not in my favor, since it was dangerously near the end of the semester and Little Napoleon hadn't yet called on me at all. If good fortune could not help me avoid his attack, then my body would have to give me the break I needed. I had no choice but to plead with my heart, the part of me that I couldn't control.

Please, heart, I begged, *let me have twenty minutes of peace. Give me this one, would you?*

My heart said no.

It was time for me to get out of that classroom; even if it meant setting myself up for the nasty nip at the heels that would come from Little Napoleon on my way out. "So nice of you to join us for a spell," he said. I was down the spiral staircase and over to the bank of pay phones before the sound of chuckling classmates faded from consciousness. Then it sank in: my heart just forced me to run out of class! I'm in the middle of an emergency! And at the same time, my mind held on to the most mundane of thoughts: I left a can of Dr Pepper on my desk—open, with a straw sticking out.

The strange thing about watching yourself in crisis is the way that the most banal thoughts can move to the forefront. As I dialed Dr. Bradley's number with shaking hands, I thought about the soda I'd left behind in the classroom and wondered how it was going to make its way to the garbage pail. Even as I described for him the heart sensations I felt—like there were popcorn kernels exploding against the inside of my chest wall—I couldn't help but notice the terrific shine on the marble floor that ran the length of the telephone vestibule. *What a well-kept law school*, I thought. *What a beautiful place*. And when I heard Dr. Bradley reply that he wanted me to come into the office and have a Holter monitor attached to my chest—a portable EKG device that would give him a twenty-four-hour reading of my heart rhythms—and a friend passed by and mouthed silently, *Pretty sweater! New?* I managed to enjoy the compliment some, even as I continued to feel the crazy sequences of heartbeats running along my insides like skipping stones: *beat . . . beat-beat . . . beat-beat-beat . . . splash!* In spite of these heart rhythms that squeezed the expanse of my breathing into miniature gasps, life around me continued in full swing. Even my own life went on.

Medical emergencies—I would learn on that day—do not cause the more ordinary aspects of life to disappear; not even for a moment. For very sick people like me, the unimaginable gets played out right alongside the completely familiar. And sometimes it is the memory of the small benign details, rather than the scary big picture, that has staying power. The prevailing image of the soda can would prevent me from drinking even one sip of Dr Pepper ever again. Many other ordinary but revealing symbols would set in my memory as well, each one a representation of what a sick heart can do to the person who must carry it around in her chest and beg its mercy. One of these was a butter-yellow skirt and matching jacket, along with a chunky string of pearls: the outfit I had bought especially for Scott's law school graduation. I had slung it over the back of his desk chair on the night before the ceremony and never saw it again.

This abandoned graduation outfit came to mind more than once—with a stomach-turning sense of loss—as Scott raced me to the hospital, the screeching tires of his car sounding an alarm of urgency around corners and through the narrow streets of Philadelphia.

It was mid-May and Scott was graduating from Penn Law School with high honors. His parents were to arrive the next morning, along with his two older brothers, just in time for the ceremony. I had arrived in Philadelphia on my usual Friday-night train with the yellow suit folded carefully into my overnight bag. The minute I arrived at Scott's apartment, I unpacked everything before too many wrinkles set in. Seeing that there was barely an extra hanger in the closet, I draped the outfit over a chair, expecting to slip into it the following morning.

But first there was dinner; we always ate out on Friday nights. Scott began listing restaurant options by type of cuisine: we could do Italian, Japanese, or maybe Indian, for a change. I hid from him the fact that I could do without dinner; I'd been fighting nausea for the past couple of weeks and my appetite had decreased. Just a few days earlier, when I had worn the Holter monitor prescribed by Dr. Bradley, I had come close to throwing up. When I returned the monitor to his office for analysis, I told the nurse that I had been feeling very nauseated, and she suggested that it might be part of the stomach bug that was going around. I asked if she would please let the doctor know that I was feeling sick to my stomach, and she said she would. He was going to be calling me in a day or two anyway with the Holter monitor results; we could discuss my stomach trouble then, if it hadn't already subsided. But nearly a week had passed and Dr. Bradley had not called me, and the nausea had only gotten worse. I made the novice-patient mistake of assuming that my Holter monitor results must have been just fine—otherwise Dr. Bradley would have contacted me, right? This assumption allowed me to believe that my stomach trouble must have been coming from a virus and not from my heart, for goodness' sake.

I told Scott that Japanese sounded terrific.

More than any other memory from our dinner out that night, the image of my water glass sticks in my mind. I remember the way I kept reaching for it repeatedly; taking little sips that I hoped would calm the fluttering in my chest. Toward the end of the meal, my sick heart began making its troublesome presence known in a more forceful way by skipping beats and then pounding wildly to make up for what it had missed. I took a sip of ice water from the tall glass that sat just above the right corner of my place mat. Then there was another arrhythmic beat—more like a profound throb. And then another. I lifted my glass and took a shallow phantom sip.

Scott continued to make conversation. I smiled at him and feigned interest. Then there was a lull and it was my turn to introduce a new topic; I began a sentence about an acquaintance of ours that I'd run into recently; a heartbeat stopped me. But this was just the beginning; apparently this one beat threw my heart into a whole new rhythm—one that I knew right away was different and terrible. This was ventricular fibrillation, the killer that had finally arrived in full force after months of teasing me with small showings of its arrhythmic power.

I tried one more sip of water but couldn't swallow. I spit it out onto my plate.

"Scotty, I don't feel right."

I'd never said anything like this to him before. Over the months that I had lived with the diagnosis of a heart virus on the mend, Scott and I had never known an emergency situation together. I had been through a couple of them on my own—my mind only half aware and clouded by optimism that allowed me to plow forward—but I'd never reached the point where I called out for help. And even on this night, I didn't really call out; I just made a statement as serenely as I could, given the water and spit that now glistened on my empty plate.

Scott wasn't buying my calm demeanor for one minute.

"I'm taking you to the hospital," he said. He paid the check in a flash on our way out the door and held me tight by the arm until we reached the parking lot.

In later years, Scott would recount this night for me with details of our dash to the hospital. "I was up on curbs—driving on the sidewalks. I nearly bottomed out my car—do you remember? I didn't know where the hospital was exactly, so I drove like a wild man. I made turns like you wouldn't believe."

For Scott, it was the frantic maneuvering of his car that he would remember most—the way his Toyota rattled as it came down hard from the edge of a curb. There was also, of course, the way I sat in the passenger's seat beside him—leaning forward, chest to knees, calling out in breathy desperation, "This is very bad. Hospital, hospital. Go faster." I would not recall bumping up against any curbs. For me, the short ride to the hospital contained a vivid image of Scott's denim-covered right thigh and the way I gripped it tight with the fingers of my left hand. I remained locked in this position until the car came to a screeching halt. Never again would I allow myself to place my hand on Scott's leg while he was driving. There was a memory in it I couldn't bear: a car ride that delivered me from the wait-and-see realm of a person with a heart condition into the chaotic moment of a true cardiac emergency.

"How old are you! Did you take any drugs tonight! Any drinking! Are you allergic to any medications!" One of the white-coated people was barking questions at me while another was cutting off my skirt with an industrial size pair of scissors. I heard the rip of soft cotton as my favorite skirt fell away from my body; and then my shirt slid off as well, having been split up the middle.

"Cardiomyopathy," I said, between gasps. "Dr. Bradley. New York Hospital. No drugs, no alcohol. Penicillin allergy. Twenty-four." Then I listed my medications in breathy whispers. There was a white coat on my left side forcing an IV needle into the top of my hand and another one sticking EKG leads on my chest and arms. No less than five people circled around my stretcher, all with urgent tasks to accomplish in little time.

"We've got a line!" someone called out. This meant that the IV was in place and ready to release antiarrhythmia drugs into my bloodstream.

Then pandemonium. Once the steady picture of my EKG appeared on the screen above my head, it was obvious to the doctors that there was no time for a slow IV drip; they needed to save my life right away. Not only was my heart showing the dangerous rhythm of ventricular fibrillation, it also revealed a severe degree of muscle damage. I would need to be defibrillated immediately. The doctors could only hope that my failing heart would be strong enough to respond well to a defibrillator shock to the chest and pop back into a rhythm that would be—at best—less lethal than the V-fib I was in. They didn't have any expectation of being able to restore total normalcy—not to this heart.

I saw two pads—defibrillator paddles, as I would later learn to call them, correctly—coming toward my chest. The sound of my own words echoed back at me as if they were coming from someone else, and I was terrified by what I heard: "Don't let me die! I love my Scotty. I love my Scotty. . . ."

And there he was—my Scotty—down at the far end of the stretcher, holding my toes. No one had asked him to leave the room, so he stayed there with me and became a reluctant witness to a gruesome sight that would be his alone to remember for all time; I would know it only by the defibrillator burn marks that showed up on my chest the next day as reddish outlines in the shape of the undersides of a pair of children's shoes. Scott had looked on as the searing electric shock came rushing through the paddles and into my chest, lifting my body off the stretcher and then dropping it down again—twice—so that a more normal heart rhythm could be restored. He would tell me later that I had been awake during those shocks; my eyes had been open the whole time. But I would have no memory of it because of the effects of a lovely intravenous drug called Versed, which was released through my IV in perfect timing with the arrival of the defibrillator paddles. I would encounter this drug on many terrifying occasions in the future—so many times, in fact, that I would come to give it a nickname: the forgetting drug. Versed took away memories or, better still, prevented them from forming to begin with. It was an important intravenous wonder drug to have on hand for a heart patient who came up against defibrillator paddles with intolerable regularity.

But the timing was such that Versed only worked to erase the middle parts of my near-death experiences. Everything that happened before and after the defibrillator shocks stayed with me. I would know what it is like to be fully aware and alert in the moment when the line between life and death becomes whisper thin. I would understand the nightmare of powerlessness; at the foot of my stretcher stood a love that I tried to hold on to with all the strength I had left, but my failing heart pulled me toward death and all I could do was call out, "Save me!" The Versed did not arrive in time to spare me the memory of how it felt to lose all control over my body—and this was really too bad.

7

"YOU'RE A VERY SICK GIRL, AMY."

These were the last words Dr. Bradley would ever say to me. He said them quietly, though not reluctantly, in response to the question I spat at him in anger and dismay: "What's going on here?"

It was the morning after my first attack of ventricular fibrillation, and I called Dr. Bradley from a bedside phone in my Philadelphia hospital room. He'd been in contact with the emergency room doctors several times overnight and knew full well that my heart failure had taken a very bad turn. But instead of explaining what had happened to me, he chose to answer my question as if merely pointing out the obvious: I was a very sick girl. Didn't I know?

No, I didn't. I thought I had four or five more months of wait-and-see time still coming to me. I wasn't supposed to get really sick yet. And I certainly wasn't supposed to have a sudden attack. It felt like I'd been duped.

My anger was instant. "What kind of doctor are you anyway?!"

Scott's reproachful glare tugged at me from across the room. He would not accept this yelling at my doctor. Dr. Bradley hadn't done anything wrong; it was just a difficult situation. I needed to be nicer—much nicer—and hold my tongue.

"You're a terrible doctor, that's what you are!"

Scott approached my bedside and wrapped his fingers around the coil of cord that ran from the base of the telephone to the receiver, a signal that it was time for me to end the call. I sped up my shouting and managed to get in a few more choice words—including "Fool!" "Idiot!" and "Liar!"—before passing the phone to Scott, who placed it back on the night table. He sat down on the side of my bed.

"You're angry with me," I said, struggling to recover my breath.

"I'm not." He reached toward my face and adjusted the oxygen tubes that had gone askew beneath my nostrils.

"You're missing out on your law school graduation right at this very moment, all because of me!"

"It's not your fault."

"It is. I've ruined your graduation."

"No, you haven't."

"Your whole family came to Philadelphia for nothing!"

"It's okay, really."

Scott could have gone on and on like this, effortlessly demonstrating the kindness he so wanted me to extend to others. He touched my cheek lightly with the back of his hand and smiled. "I want to be here with you. You're my girl," he said.

"I'm your sick girl."

It was the first time I'd said it. Scott brushed my silliness away with a kiss on my forehead and changed the subject. But he didn't know that Dr. Bradley had just assigned a new label to me, one that would settle in place for all time, like cement. "Sick girl" held more meaning for me than the medical term *cardiomyopathy* ever could, and it would prove more damaging. Dr. Bradley's words on that morning were to echo through my life and creep into every thought I would ever have about myself: I am a lawyer—*but I am a sick girl;* it's the tenth anniversary of my heart transplant—*but I am a sick girl;* Scott is the love of my life—*but I am a sick girl.*

I lost the battle against this pithy label, to be sure. But I did not give in without first questioning the doctor who'd thrown it at me without warning. From the moment I hung up the phone on that Philadelphia morning—in haste and under Scott's critical gaze—I knew I was not yet done with Dr. Bradley.

I decided to write this slippery eel a letter as soon as possible. A hospital social worker with a syrupy sweetness was eager to help me slide this one by. She brought writing paper, pen, and a stamped envelope to my bedside on the double—the perky dear—so I could "get it all out," she said, sure that the exercise of writing would be a "super healthy release" for my feelings.

My letter to Dr. Bradley began with the super-healthy release of a bitter accusation couched in a direct question: "When did you start lying to me?"

I couldn't tell for sure when and how the deceit had begun. There certainly were no clues in the handwritten note I received back from Dr. Bradley a few days later. Every sentence in his short reply reeked of a lawyer's careful scrutiny; he said things like "Illness can make people feel angry and very sad—it can make them want to lash out and blame someone, even when there is no one to blame." But I hadn't blamed Dr. Bradley for my illness; I only faulted him for hiding it from me. And now he'd given me reason to believe that, somewhere along the line, his protective disclosure had turned into flat-out lying. It had taken a lethal attack of ventricular fibrillation to force the moment of truth on both of us—me and my evasive cardiologist.

"How'd that letter go?" The social worker was back again the next day. She stood just outside my room, so that most of her body was hidden, and then popped her head into view with a cluck and a wink. Then she took a sprightly hop to the right and bounced herself into the middle of the open doorway. The singsong greeting and clownish leap had failed to charm me, and she was compelled to do what any respectable professional with an ulterior motive like hers would do: reach into her counseling bag of tricks and pull out an irresistible lure.

Her cheerful smile collapsed at once into the close-mouthed grin of an alley cat. She moved toward my bed in slow small steps purring the words she knew would interest me. There was an important message from the docs downstairs, she said. Would I like to hear it now, or should she come back at a better time?

"Does it have anything to do with getting me out of here and back to New York?"

"Well, yes, it does! You're really on top of things, I see. Isn't that just so terrific?" she purred.

It took self-control not to let my repulsion show.

She finally delivered her message. The doctors preferred to stay in the shadows on the messy issue of my hospital discharge. There was, apparently, a lot at stake in the timing of my departure from the hospital. It had already been decided that I needed to return to New York and be admitted to Columbia-Presbyterian Hospital. It had also been determined that my heart rhythm was much too unstable for me to travel by car or train, so I would have to be transported by ambulance, with an experienced cardiologist and a defibrillator on board. The only question that remained was how soon I would leave Philadelphia. At this point, the question was no longer medical; it was one of preference, and the answer was up to me.

"It's no secret that your heart problem is more than we can handle," the social worker said, having regained some of her calm. We're a small suburban hospital, and we can't make you better here. We can only be a bridge for you on your journey.

"But we're also a teaching hospital, and a heart like yours can certainly do a lot of teaching. The docs wanted me to let you know that they understand if you choose to go to Columbia right away. But they'd be so pleased if you'd agree to stay here for a few more days so they can share your case with the medical students. It's tremendously interesting. Really instructive. Maybe you'd consider helping us out—just for a day or two more."

So the doctors who saved my life with a defibrillator in the emergency room were now asking me to return the favor. They'd snatched me from jaws of danger just a few days earlier—and continued to be at the ready to do so again and again—and I was now forced to decide whether or not to grant them this little request. Just a couple of days more at this small hospital, all for the sake of advancing the knowledge of specialists and their wide-eyed students who'd never seen anything like me; that's all they were asking. These were the people who had saved my life, after all. The least I could do was share my heart with them for a little while longer.

And what if I said no? Would they run into my room and save me from V-fib tonight just as quickly as they had before, and with the same intensity and resolve? Or would they figure I was an ungrateful patient who was not willing to share her fascinating heart with the very people who'd kept it beating, and therefore my life wasn't worth saving all that much. They sure would be able to take a good close look at my heart once I was dead, wouldn't they? I would make a terrific cadaver for an autopsy class.

"The docs said you can take your time deciding. No pressure," the social worker said.

I told her I needed no time at all. I was going to Columbia as soon as possible: tomorrow morning, if it could be arranged. I was getting the hell out of Philadelphia before the doctors let me die here—in the interests of medical education, of course.

8

WITH A DEPARTURE AS ABRUPT AS MINE, IT COULDN'T BE AVOIDED: pieces of my life got left behind in Philadelphia. Some of them I knew full well I was leaving there, like my overnight bag and the three study outlines I'd already prepared for upcoming final exams. Other things were less apparent—losses I could not have anticipated.

Like, for instance, showers. I'd taken a quick one at Scott's apartment just before we went out for that fateful dinner at the Japanese restaurant. I didn't know at the time—or even days later, during my ambulance ride to New York—that I would leave the pleasant routine of showering behind me. I had no sense as I stepped over the edge of the tub and onto the bath mat that I would not be able to take a shower or wash my hair again for two whole months. Within a week of leaving Philadelphia, the motion of lifting a handful of shampoo up to my head and working it into a lather (which, previously, had been effortless) came close to setting off a punishing episode of V-fib, even before I had time to rinse out the suds. Sponge baths quickly became the order of the day.

Then there was fresh air; I'd left this behind as well. As two hospital workers maneuvered my stretcher through the emergency room doors, out to the hospital parking area, and quickly into the back of a waiting ambulance, the oxygen tubes fell away from my nose for a moment and I inhaled the warm spring air without particular awareness. There was nothing in the fifteen seconds between door and ambulance that suggested to me that I should savor these outdoor breaths because they might be the last ones I would take for a long, long time. The windows in my hospital room in New York City, as it turned out, wouldn't open; nor would the one tiny faux window in the Intensive Care Unit cubicle where I was to spend the greater part of my hospital stay. For what seemed like an eternity, I would be surrounded by the stale, recirculated, ammonia-tinged air of Columbia-Presbyterian Hospital, and I could only escape it by closing my eyes and trying hard to recall the feeling of a soft breeze. It would be two slow treacherous months before I would be able to step outside again and take another breath.

No one anticipated that my hospital stay at Columbia would last that long—least of all my new cardiologist, Dr. Ganz. He came to my bedside soon after I settled into my unfamiliar surroundings and told me, matter-of-factly, that we were going to get to the bottom of this *arrhythmia* problem of mine. He didn't say the words heart failure, and I took this as a positive sign. Something terrible had certainly happened to me back there in Philadelphia, but whatever it was seemed to have narrowed the scope of my cardiac problem into a more discrete issue, and this could only be good. Now my heart condition had a name that made sense to me. I didn't need to bother guessing anymore at what the strange term *cardiomyopathy* meant and how it might feel in my body. Now I had a new illness with a new cardiac specialist to match, and I hoped that both of these might prove to be the most patient-friendly yet.

It was just the sort of nudge I needed to start thinking more positively again—even in the wake of V-fib. I allowed myself to nibble at the happy thought that sometimes things have to get worse before they get better. Maybe the defibrillator paddles had been the beginning of a step in the right direction. Perhaps this new condition of mine, arrhythmia, which Dr. Ganz had just detailed for me with a reassuring absence of alarm, wasn't such a big deal after all. He told me there were a number of things that could be done to correct the problem, and we were going to begin with the most simple among them: medication. That made sense to me, didn't it? I was on board with that?

He paused politely after each sentence, just to make sure we were in agreement before he moved on.

I should know, he said, that he'd already made arrangements for a diagnostic test that would help target just the right anti-arrhythmia drug to protect my heart from slipping into V-fib. He hoped this was all right with me. The test would be uncomfortable—not an easy exam by any means—but one that was absolutely necessary to fine-tune my medication. We were going to start as soon as possible. Get things under control so I could go home. How did that sound?

"I'm sure you don't want to hang around here any longer than you have to," he said, "although I hear the food's not too bad!" He winked at me and then flashed a honey grin at the hospital aide who'd just placed my lunch tray down. She smiled back at him. I surprised myself and did the same: smiled spontaneously at a doctor!

What a nice guy. And he seemed to have some good news for me—or maybe it was just Dr. Ganz himself that was the good news. Everything about him was a comfort to me, from the deep tone of assuredness that hummed beneath his words to his perfectly knotted, stylish tie that pulled my attention away from the white doctor's coat that lay ominously on either side of it. He stood over my bed, a graceful palm tree, all six-foot-something of him, and looked directly at me with eyes that were so calming, so unusually genuine, that they seemed to lift my body out of the hospital bed and suspend it right up alongside him—eye to eye—so that I could, for the first time, know what it was like to be on the same level with my own doctor. I was not a twenty-four-year-old child as I floated up there beside Dr. Ganz. I wasn't a crazy patient either. I wasn't even a very sick girl. I was—for a brief moment—myself again.

And maybe—just maybe—there was hope.

"You know what?" he chimed, with a playful wave in the direction of the IV fluid bag hanging beside me, "we can get rid of those meds the doctors started you on in Philadelphia. We'll stop them right now. Then tomorrow morning you can go in for the test without any antiarrhythmia medicine in your bloodstream, and we'll find out just what you need, all right?" He paused, awaiting my answer, and in the few seconds that it took for me to nod my head yes, the expression on his face changed from kindly to solemn. "Good. See you tomorrow then. But meanwhile, please—and I mean this—let me know if there is anything I can do for you."

He held his right hand out for me to shake. When I gave him mine in return, he placed his left hand directly on top and held it there. Then he repeated the offer a second time, bringing it right into the present moment as proof of his earnestness. "Is there something I can do for you now, before I go?"

A few options ran through my mind: *Another blanket? A softer pillow? Maybe he could find me a radio so I could listen to some music. . . .*

"Any questions? Concerns?" he asked, still urging me on with soft-spoken insistence. If I had any, they didn't seem all that important now that Dr. Ganz was holding my hand in that wonderful cocoon of reassurance he'd created between his own.

In the days, months, and years that followed, I would look back on this moment of handholding and wonder how things might have turned out if I hadn't let myself become so taken by this truly lovely fellow, my new doctor. Why didn't I act like a smart patient? It was a lesson I still hadn't learned: a smart patient will always maintain a safe level of doubt no matter how kindly, earnest, or intelligent her doctor may be. There was a price to be paid for dumbing myself down, for allowing a gentle smile and a lingering handshake to stifle my intuition and inquisitiveness. As my punishment, it seemed, I would be plagued by thoughts of what I should have said and what I actually had said when Dr. Ganz opened the door to my input with all graciousness and welcome. I'd told him, "No, thanks, I'm fine."

What a mistake.

The next morning, Scott was in my hospital room, having arrived early with my breakfast: a bagel and juice. After just a few bites, an odd sensation rose up in my chest; it seemed to be coming from my stomach. There was a little kick, and then another one, and then a series of them: *kick-kick-kick-kick.*

I stopped in the middle of a sentence and brought my hands to my abdomen. Scott gave me a questioning look. "My stomach," I said. "It's bumping around. I don't know—"

"I'm sure it's nothing," he said, gathering up the remains of the bagel I still held in my lap. He placed them on the night table and motioned for me to scoot over in the bed. "Enough of this breakfast. I'm comin' in for a hug—"

He had one knee up on the mattress when the alarm wailed.

Until that moment, neither Scott nor I had noticed—right up there above my door—an innocent-looking circular knob sticking out of the wall. But now it was flashing red and blasting as loud as a fire engine. Somehow this alarm had figured out that the stomach bumps were actually coming from my heart. I looked back over my shoulder at the EKG screen and realized the connection at once: the alarm must have been tripped by the information flowing from the EKG leads on my chest to the monitor behind me. My heartbeat had been under constant observation, and I hadn't even known it.

Did I really need to be watched this closely?

I lay back on the pillow and began my desperate self-cure at once, singing out the first melody that came to mind. Meanwhile, a crowd had formed just outside the door. My nurse was the first one through. He looked up at the lines on the EKG monitor and plunged the end of his stethoscope beneath my hospital gown without moving his eyes from the screen. His other hand shot up in front of my face. "Shhh! Shhh!"

I had to stop singing.

"It's just my stomach, don't you think, Fred?"

"Shhh. . . ."

"You feel bumps sometimes after you eat, right, Fred?"

"Oh, I don't know. . . ."

He shifted his glance away from the monitor and signaled to Scott by lifting his eyebrows up twice. As Scott retreated dutifully to the corner of the room, doctors and nurses began to file in—some in a hurry to reach me, others less urgent, sauntering their way into a horseshoe shape at the end of my hospital bed. Now, it seemed, I had the beginnings of an audience, which would continue to grow by the minute; my heartbeat was once again about to become a show. Scott remained at the far end of my room, slowly disappearing behind the expanding mass of white coats.

"Scotty! Don't leave me!"

"I'm right here. I'm not going anywhere," he said, stepping back into view. "Look at me. Just look. Here I am."

Scott was smiling. He had his hand up in the air, waving casually.

The IV pole rattled beside my bed as a nurse tossed a bag of antiarrhythmia medicine onto the metal hook. Scott managed to hold on to his smile—every feature of his face reaching out to me so that I could feel his steady presence, his encouragement—even though he knew what was coming next. He had witnessed it before. Scott and I would ride out this episode of V-fib together—and just barely.

"Damn!"

The doctor in charge—whom I had never met—began to pace back and forth at the foot of my bed. He lifted his hands up and down, up and down, in a sort of what-are-we-to-do? motion, and then burst out again—this time, even louder—"Damn!"

He had just ordered a quick intravenous blast of antiarrhythmia medication—a reintroduction of the same drug Dr. Ganz had stopped the night before—but my heartbeat continued to race right through it, completely undaunted. The medicine wasn't working.

"Let's get the next one going—now!"

Again, the clattering of the IV pole as a nurse tossed on another bag of medicine. I turned my head to the side and saw the doctor standing in front of the EKG monitor, his thumb and pointer finger spread across his forehead as if he were looking into direct sunlight. He winced, and down came his right hand—*slap*—against his thigh.

"Oh, come on!" he shouted, spinning away from the EKG reading that had just let him know that the second medication was failing as well. He flew into a three-quarter turn and came to a sudden stop at my bedside: feet set wide apart, body leaning forward, arms bent at the elbows. Fat beads of sweat had broken out on his forehead; one of them dropped to the tip of his nose and then fell as the corners of his mouth pulled back into the shape of a silent growl. This man didn't look much like a doctor to me anymore, even with his long white coat and stethoscope hanging down from his neck. This was an angry man ready for a fight.

Was I his enemy? Or was it my heart?

He lifted his troubled gaze from the floor and brought it to rest at the top of my forehead, ignoring the entreaty from my own eyes just inches below. Staring at my hairline as if into a black hole, my doctor made it clear just whom—or what—he was fighting against; it was my heart that was his adversary, of course. This doctor couldn't possibly be angry with me, because I, Amy—the law student, the young woman, the whole person—wasn't there anymore. His blank stare told me so. It confirmed that I had left myself behind in Philadelphia, sitting at a table in front of a half-eaten tray of sushi. Sure, my body had gotten up and walked away from that table, but the rest of me had remained seated there: my sense of self, my sense of peace, and the fundamental sense that there was so much more to me than just my heart, sick or well. On this morning and for the next two months that I would spend in the hospital, there would be a new Amy forced upon me, and this diluted self could only be seen in the frightfully abnormal lines running across the EKG monitor. These lines revealed the most severe disease, the most precarious rhythms that teetered on the verge of V-fib and caused endless problems for the medical staff. No doctor or nurse could walk into my room and greet me without first pausing in front of the EKG screen and staring—in obvious horror. My heart was ugly. It was bad. It was disgustingly sick.

And it was me.

I wanted to scream out, *I hate my own heart!* But I couldn't do it; my breath was nearly gone.

The antiarrhythmia medicines having failed to stop the V-fib by now, a defibrillator cart roared up alongside me. The doctor reached for the paddles and I turned my head away from him, bringing it back to center. Now all I had was the perfect square of white ceiling above my hospital bed to tell me my fate. I looked up at it and felt imminent powerlessness pressing down on me, just as it had in Philadelphia. I knew I had no time to lose; if I was going to do something—anything—it had to be this very minute. It would take every bit of my strength, but I would use whatever I had left so that I might perform one final act of will, one last exercise of self-control. With eyes wide open and full of courageous intent, I summoned up the power and did it: I surrendered—to death, to being saved, to the doctor's anger, and to the defibrillator paddles that lay at the ready, flat against my chest. There was no use fighting, no use singing. And even if I were able to call out a final impassioned plea, "Save me! Please!" it wouldn't make any difference. My life—or death—all came down to the beating of my sick heart, whose perilous rhythm wouldn't listen to me. And it seemed to be giving this sweaty, struggling cardiologist a terrible time, resisting him at every turn, thrashing about like a six-foot marlin hooked straight through the mouth.

The doctor counted, "Three, two, one!" and the electricity surged. The battle was on.

Bam! A shock ran through me; it grabbed my body by the breastbone, lifted it up, and threw it down as if from the window of a tall building. My hospital bed evaporated and I landed—*splat*—a free-fallen nightmare on a slab of reality-splintering cement.

The room was silent as everyone paused to see if a change in my heart rhythm would appear on the screen. It didn't. The V-fib continued with a vengeance. The punishing jolts of electricity had only intensified the erratic starts and stops pounding against my chest wall. I took in a slow breath as best I could, let it out, and then froze—not by choice. Deathly arrhythmia had finally stolen away the air.

Through a haze of semiconsciousness, I heard the doctor shout out, "We're losing her!"

Even without breath, I knew in an instant that he was wrong. The doctors and nurses weren't losing me. They were losing my heart. That was all.

I felt the defibrillator panels cool against my skin for the second time. Another shock was on the way and there was nothing I could do about it.

The doctor began again, "Three, two, one!"

"I love my Scotty," I mumbled, and passed out.

9

TWO DAYS LATER, I LAY ON A TABLE AWAITING THE DIAGNOSTIC TEST Dr. Ganz had promised, which had been put off by the unexpected episode of V-fib. This time he decided not to take me off arrhythmia medicine prior to the exam.

A nurse stood beside me. "Cold and wet—on the way!" she chirped.

This was a friendly warning. A sterile wash was about to be applied to a tingling patch of freshly shaved skin on the right side of my groin. The nurse held the dripping wet gauze with scissor tongs and swabbed a good portion of my hip, thigh, and abdomen, paying special attention to the soft spot just beneath the right side of my pubic bone. I appreciated the advance notice; the icy wetness sent a shiver through me—plus, it stung.

"*Ay, ay!*"

"*Ay?* Looks like we've got Ricky Ricardo with us this morning, folks!" The nurse sidestepped her way to the top of the exam table until she reached my shoulders. She smiled down at me, "You remember *I Love Lucy,* don't you?"

A doctor approached with a clipboard and pen in hand. It was time for me to sign a consent form. I hadn't been asked to sign one since the biopsy and angiogram seven months earlier when I was Dr. Bradley's patient. I cast my eyes down and allowed my mind to wander while the doctor rattled off some gruesome possibilities that I would have no choice but to accept with a reluctant signature at the bottom of the page. There was no reason for me to listen closely to this doctor's recitations; Dr. Ganz had already explained everything to me. This electrophysiology test sounded like a fairly straightforward diagnostic exam; it would allow the doctor to pinpoint exactly the medication that would work best to protect me from future episodes of V-fib.

This exam was going to seem familiar to me in some ways, Dr. Ganz had said. It would be a sort of biopsy/angiogram combination—nothing I couldn't handle. A catheter would be inserted into my groin and maneuvered up into my heart, where it would tickle its way around and induce an arrhythmia on purpose. A doctor would then release a particular antiarrhythmia medication into my bloodstream intravenously. If this medicine didn't work to correct my heart rhythm, the doctor would remove the stimulus of the arrhythmia (the tickling catheter) and my heartbeat would return to normal on its own. Then the whole procedure could be repeated again and again, if necessary, until an effective antiarrhythmia drug could be identified. It was a bit of trial and error. But Dr. Ganz was still hopeful that there would be a medical (as opposed to surgical) solution to my arrhythmia problem and that the electrophysiology test would lead us to it.

I signed the consent form.

Then came the first probe of the catheter. It bumped up against my heart, eliciting arrhythmia. I welcomed the first couple of offbeats, knowing that the procedure was moving along as Dr. Ganz had told me it would.

"I feel something," I said.

"Yes, we know." They could see it on the EKG. Powerful medication was already on its way to my heart.

"But now I feel dizzy." It had never hit me so hard and fast during an arrhythmia attack before.

The doctor quickly pulled back on the catheter, expecting that my heartbeat would settle down. But instead, it just stopped.

My heart. Stopped. And my breathing. Stopped.

The telltale flatline appeared up on the screen. I was "dead."

This is the point where I was supposed to go through a long tunnel or take spirit form and float above the scene of my body. Flatliners like me have reported seeing their lives flash before them, like images outside the window of a speeding train: birthday parties, graduations, and wedding ceremonies, all in bold details that soften and blur immediately upon recognition. Other people have told of the sense of being escorted on a journey—beyond their will but comforting just the same—guided by an invisible force they trust completely. Some have even seen family members who are already dead or beloved pets they lost years before. The stories vary a bit from person to person, but what they all have in common is the presence of light; there is a bright, warm, welcoming light that draws them in with such tenderness and calm that there is no more fear, no more pain, and no more worry. Wherever the person may be headed, it is a good place—a perfect place, even. And at the moment when it becomes apparent that somehow the direction has been changed and their body has actually begun to move away from the light, there is sadness in the recognition that a return to the earthly world is at hand. But at the same time, there is joy—because the light remains. When the person comes back, he or she will keep forever the illumination of knowing that there is someplace we go after death, and that this place is peaceful, safe, and brighter than anything we've ever seen: whiter than white.

But I saw only black.

The dizziness was brief, and it ended me. One moment I was there, and the next I was not. It was like all the nights in my life when I'd get into bed, close my eyes, anticipate sleep, and not realize that that sleep had come to me until I woke in the morning. Like sleep, death is something you slip into unaware. It is without sight or sound. It is without fanfare. And it is most definitely without light. Death is darkness. That is all.

There is trauma in knowing this: experiencing something that is not supposed to be experienced, knowing something that is better left unknown. I would carry with me the memory of what I perceived (and what the monitors of my vital signs confirmed) as death—and it was nothingness. For me, the end of life had revealed itself to be no big deal and certainly no celebration. No one would ever be willing to take my word for it and live with this idea in mind; what I witnessed on the electrophysiology table that day set me apart from most people I knew. And that's how the trauma of my arrhythmia attacks chipped away at me: I lived every day with the unshakable and unpopular belief that death was permanent darkness.

There were those who tried to convince me otherwise. They urged me to consider that maybe I didn't see the light because it wasn't my time to die. Or that maybe the tunnel was there and I was in it but I didn't remember. But neither of these made sense to me. I could only shake my head and say with conviction and apology, "I know what I know, and I couldn't be more sure of it. Death is nothingness. Sorry."

Only life is full of light, color, and sensation.

I felt it come back to me immediately when I opened my eyes in the electrophysiology suite. I'd left this room behind just minutes before, and now here it was again, just as I remembered it. Except that one of the nurses appeared to be crying and repeating my name over and over, "Amy! Amy! Amy!"

"Here I am," I said, opening my eyes, not sure what I was waking from. The nurse put her hand to her chest and exhaled.

I heard a doctor say, "Good. That's fine now. Let's get her back to the ICU." The exam room became very busy. Everyone seemed in a rush to tidy up, reset the machinery, and prepare my stretcher for a trip down the hall. Was that why no one slowed down to speak with me for a moment? I hadn't yet heard anything about whether they'd found a medical solution to my arrhythmia.

The nurse wheeled my stretcher out of the exam room. Dr. Ganz appeared out of nowhere.

I looked up at him with a smile. "Can I have my breakfast now? I'm starved."

"Of course, sure. We've got to talk first, though. I've invited your father in, okay?"

I tilted my head up and saw my father standing by the door, his arms hanging down in front of his body, hands clasped. Dr. Ganz reached forward and adjusted the top portion of my stretcher so I could sit up a bit. Then he leaned his hip onto the space of mattress beside me and took my hand between both of his, just like he'd done before.

"You failed the test."

"How's that?"

Dr. Ganz looked over his shoulder at my father, then turned back and brought his chin to his chest. "Your heart stopped. The medicine didn't work. I don't think any medicine is going to work."

My father stepped forward and came to a stop just behind Dr. Ganz. He unclasped his hands and let the fingers rest on my stretcher. "Amy, at this point, the doctor says. . . ."

His bottom lip began to quiver.

Dr. Ganz helped him along. "You need to have a heart transplant."

"I won't do it." My answer shot out like a bullet.

"There really isn't any other option. The test confirmed it for us," Dr. Ganz said. "We can get the paperwork going so that you'll be on the transplant list in just a few days."

The same transplant list the doctor in Boston said I didn't need to be on?

"I said I won't do it!" I lifted my shoulders completely off the pillow and yelled at my gentle doctor.

My father moved in closer, and Dr. Ganz made room for him, retreating to the wall for a moment. "Amy, honey," my father began again, shakily, "you really need to do this. . . ."

"Well, I won't. I'm not letting them cut my heart out."

Suddenly, my father's head and shoulders collapsed, dropping several feet so that his chin came to rest just above the padding on my stretcher.

My father had fallen to his knees.

"Amy, please," he said, each word a shuddering exhalation of grief, "you have to do it. You just have to. You can't leave me, Amy. Please."

My father was weeping at my bedside. I felt desperate to escape his anguish at that moment, just the way he had been driven to escape mine when he fled from the taxi in Boston. The only difference was that I couldn't get up and run; I couldn't slam the door on my father's pain the way he'd done to mine. As I lay there, prisoner to a hospital stretcher, there was only one surefire way for me to shut off the torment and I jumped at it immediately, just as quickly as my father had jumped from the backseat of the cab: I agreed—in a second—to have a heart transplant. "Okay!"

My father rose slowly from his knees. He rubbed his eyes with the heels of his hands as he walked out of the room. Dr. Ganz stepped forward and told me I had made the right choice.

I would always wonder: did I make a choice at all?

The remaining hours of that day crept by uncomfortably. My father, Beverly, and Scott took turns sitting beside me, allowing one another a few minutes of freedom from the tension and apprehension that hung in the air of my hospital room.

The doctors' report had been devastating to all of us and left disbelief in its wake. A few hours ago, I was just a cardiac patient on her way to another diagnostic test; but I returned later as

Columbia's most recent addition to the heart transplant program. The reality was too fresh, too harsh; my looming transplant was like a communal bad dream no one in my room wanted to mention. So there was mostly silence. Some hand holding. An occasional escaped tear.

The evening came upon me and my visitors almost as a surprise —when a dinner tray arrived and signaled the six o'clock hour. It was clear to everyone that a difficult night lay ahead of me. Beverly took the lead in finding a practical way to help. Glancing around my ICU cubicle, she saw that the only accommodation was a single wooden straight-back chair. Beverly laid claim to it for the night with a firm, unwavering offer. All it had taken was my telling her I felt afraid. I had died that day on the testing table and was overwhelmed by the thought that I might die—fall back into the darkness all over again—during the night.

Scott hugged Beverly long and hard before he left. Thanked her again and again. He couldn't possibly spend that night with me at the hospital. He just couldn't.

10

My heart was not supposed to have stopped during the electrophysiology test. I could see it in the way Dr. Ganz hung his head during our first moments together in the ICU—as if he'd just witnessed a terrible miscalculation of risk. On the evening before the exam, he had reassured me, saying that since I was to continue taking antiarrhythmia medicines overnight I would not be in any danger.

I'd believed Dr. Ganz, though it was the same upbeat spoonful he'd fed me a few days earlier when arriving at my bedside in the wake of a surprise attack of V-fib. On that morning he'd begun by saying that he was so sorry, but that really I should have been all right without any heart medication in my bloodstream for a few hours. Then he sprang into encouragement mode, urging me to forget about the episode (it had been a "fluke" occurrence anyway) and asking that I move my sights forward with optimism: my heartbeat would be just fine now that I was back on antiarrhythmia medicine. He cheerfully advised me to get my body up and active—walk the halls, do bicycle circles with my legs while lying in bed, swing my arms around. Apparently, it was more dangerous for me to lie motionless day after day; all kinds of bad things could come from inactivity, he told me, including muscle atrophy and even bedsores. Best to put all thoughts of ventricular fibrillation aside and keep moving—for good health.

And that was just what I did—until I flatlined during the electrophysiology exam. Then fear set in. It became much harder for me to believe this doctor's assurances and follow his advice, but I was not yet ready to abandon them entirely.

Dr. Ganz continued to encourage me to stay active—within the limits of my hospital floor. There was a lot of downtime between the diagnostics and paperwork that needed to be completed before I was officially on the heart transplant waiting list. Once or twice a day, Dr. Ganz would stop by my room and pester me in his amiable way to "move it" because light activity was good for me—truly. Keep busy, keep muscle tone, he said. It would help me after my transplant.

So, like a compliant patient eager to believe that safety could be found in following her doctor's advice with exactitude, I popped out of bed at regular intervals and did my little jaunts of hospital exercise, telling myself the whole time that I was doing something positive for my body. I continued in this way for about twenty-four hours and then got hit again—with an episode of V-fib from hell.

It didn't take much to set this one off. I simply got up out of bed, walked to the bathroom, and came back again—no more than twenty paces total. Then the alarm above my door began to wail and the white-coated circus arrived, same as before. Like clockwork, Dr. Ganz showed up (calm as ever, and sporting a handsome navy tie and coordinating suspenders) just moments after the messy, exasperating job of saving my life had been carried out by one of his colleagues. It struck me all of a sudden how odd it was that my abundantly competent and caring doctor—who was also a renowned arrhythmia specialist—never seemed to be around to do the saving himself. He was always somewhere else when the defibrillator cart pulled up alongside my bed. This may have been just a coincidence, or maybe Dr. Ganz stayed away on purpose so I wouldn't associate him with the chaotic uncertainty that swirled around the doctor who did the work: who would have to cross his fingers and send shocks of electricity through my body, not at all confident that it would help but hoping for the best. The doctor who ultimately saved me always seemed so unsure of himself and so disappointingly unnerved by my sick heart. If I'd seen Dr. Ganz acting this way, I couldn't possibly continue to believe in him. And if I was going to move beyond another devastating episode of V-fib, I was going to need a confident, reassuring doctor to believe in—even if it meant his keeping in the shadows when I needed him most.

Dr. Ganz looked directly into my eyes and admitted softly, almost in a murmur, how unfortunate it was that this particular episode of V-fib happened while I was on the new antiarrhythmia medications. It was just too bad and, again, he was "sorry." Then he lifted the tenor of his voice and told me with a hint of light humor that I must not let myself get lazy now; it was still important that I keep moving about—even if only with gentle exercises in bed.

Later that day, I brought my legs out from under the blanket and did some scissor kicks—ten at a time—and then rested. I brought my arms up and boxed with the air for a while. I forced myself to sit up in bed quickly and then lie back down again; then up and down several times more. It was what the doctor ordered, after all, so of course I did it . . .

Until I went into V-fib again.

And then I stopped being a good little patient who puts aside her own intuition.

Now I would disobey Dr. Ganz outright, even if he was the warmest, fuzziest doctor I'd ever known, and the most trustworthy. On the issue of exercise, I simply had to go against his wishes; I couldn't bear another defibrillator debacle, and I needed finally to step up (or lie down, as it were) and protect myself. I would spend the next two months of waiting-list time on my back in a hospital bed, barely turning from side to side, and never once getting up and out for more than a few seconds. Though embarrassed and disgusted by my own decision, I insisted that a bedpan become my bathroom, regardless of who would have to carry away my waste (often it would be Scott). I asked my nurse to create a piling of pillows so I could lay my full weight against them and maintain a semiupright position without exerting myself at all. I stopped laughing, stopped humming and whistling, even quit listening to music; these tended to make my heartbeat run fast, and who could tell where this might end up. I even stopped lifting my arm to brush my hair; there was too much danger in the long stroke from scalp to shoulder. In spite of the bird's nest tangling of my curls, the urine stains that accumulated on my bedsheets, and the atrophy slowly settling into my twenty-four-year-old muscles, I forced my body into near inertia—against the advice of my good doctor.

And the episodes of V-fib stopped. Just like that.

Ask a heart patient what the hardest part of the whole transplant experience is, from pre- to post-surgery, and the answer is likely to be: the wait. But as universally difficult as an open-ended vigil for a new heart may be, some patients will have an easier go of it—if only because the waiting turns out to be of relatively short duration for them. These patients are the fortunate ones.

In June of 1988, I was the luckiest patient on the heart transplant waiting list at Columbia. Just after me in luck was a nineteen-year-old boy named David, whose hospital room was diagonally across the hall, three doors down from mine. He had a lot of good things going for him too. First was his youth. Of course, his tender teenage years added an extra dimension of sadness and tragedy to his heart illness, but these years also boosted him high on the waiting list—very close to the top, in fact. And then there were the auspicious particulars of his heart problem: the absence of a manageable genetic heart defect and the mysterious onset of a rare and virulent cardiomyopathy, just like mine—but his was without ventricular tachycardia, which meant no defibrillator paddles. David was as sick as a boy could be, with a heart muscle that was in the most advanced stages of failure, but he wasn't having attacks of any kind and the alarm never went off above his door. Young David was simply dying—precipitously—and this was a fortunate circumstance; it necessitated that he remain in the hospital while waiting for a donor heart. Obligatory hospitalization—an enviable plus—pushed him up even further on the list.

David was one lucky guy.

For the many, many patients on the heart transplant waiting list, success is found in having the sickest heart imaginable. Better still is a heart condition that becomes progressively worse each day and proves itself to be increasingly unstoppable. End-stage heart failure—in all its tragedy and horror—is the means by which a patient climbs steadily up the ladder of transplant priority. In order to be so lifted, a patient must first plunge to the depths; those who aren't sinking fast into the quicksand of their heart disease are at a deadly disadvantage. This strange reality tends to place pretransplant patients in the prickly counterintuitive position of feeling distraught when diagnostic testing reveals a level of heart function that is only wishy-washy, middle-of-the-road bad but not quite awful—a disappointing result that can place them on the transplant waiting list but at the same time deprive them of the chance of getting a new heart anytime soon. It's a mind-bending delicate balance: the sicker you are, the more likely you are to receive what you need in order to live; but at the same time, the greater the chance is that you won't live long enough to get what you've been waiting for—the elusive gift of life that just might come at any time.

Or it might not come at all. For most patients, their great fortune in having the most serious of all heart conditions will eventually show its inherent downside and kill them before they get a new heart. There are, after all, thousands of people on heart transplant waiting lists at hospitals across the country, and only a few hundred hearts will become available through donation each year (only about half of the families approached by organ procurement specialists will agree to donate the organs of a loved one who has been pronounced brain dead). With so few hearts to go around, the waiting list becomes a game that very few will win.

Like me and David. We were winners, at the top of the game, playing with the odds in our favor: sick beyond all hope and young to boot. David had been spared the dangerous arrhythmia I battled, and this made him even luckier than I was—not because of how it affected his position on the waiting list (it didn't) but because his brushes with death were more subtle than mine and didn't involve electrical shocks to the chest. David recognized this small but vital difference in our medical situations, as shown by his response when a doctor dashed into his hospital room one afternoon and gave him the wonderful news: a donor heart had become available—for him! David was thrilled to hear it, of course, but woven into the first few sentences of his ebullient reply was a striking expression of consideration—for me. "What about Amy?" he asked the doctor. "She's sicker than I am. She should get this heart."

David had heard the alarm above my door on the many occasions it cried out for the white coats. A doctor assured him that this particular donor heart did not match his neighbor's blood type—otherwise, it would have been hers.

I was, after all, number one on the heart transplant waiting list for the New York area. It was true that David's position was somewhere below mine and it would seem fairer for me to get a heart first, but that's how things worked on the list. David's good news was the result of a careful and painstakingly objective process of selection made by an independent organ donation network. Skipping down a name or two on the list in order to achieve a matching donor/recipient blood type was a well-documented and fully rule-abiding practice.

David got his new heart fair and square.

What a joyous afternoon on the cardiac floor. The hallway echoed with unusually exuberant sounds as two operating room nurses wheeled David's stretcher to the elevator bank. Beverly poked her head outside my door and watched the procession glide by, relaying details to me in a play-by-play of David's journey down the hall: "He's sitting straight up. He's waving and smiling to everyone. Now he's giving the thumbs-up sign." David's usual pallor was gone, and in its place was a flush of healthy color—as if new life had already been pumped into him, she told me.

Lucky David. He was on his way to be saved.

"Good for him, right?" Beverly said.

Right.

Kind of.

More than a swell of happiness for my fellow patient, I felt an embarrassing twinge of envy. David had got a quick ticket out of the waiting game. And out of the hospital. He even got to be the subject of a PBS documentary about heart transplantation (a film crew followed his stretcher into the operating room). A lower number than mine on the waiting list was about to receive the precious gift of life, while I would have to remain in a hospital bed perpetually on the verge of killer V-fib, with a frighteningly unreliable antiarrhythmia cocktail pumping through my veins.

But still, I was fortunate—even with my extended waiting time.

Because David didn't live for long.

He made it through the transplant surgery well enough and went on to an uneventful and steady recovery. But within the first few years, David's transplanted heart gave out—way before expected. Sometimes new hearts do that: begin a precipitous path of self-destruction soon after transplant and slip quickly beyond saving. This kind of deterioration is the result of a phenomenon called *rejection,* the scourge of heart transplantation, where the body's immune system attacks the new heart as a foreign object. In some cases, the onset of rejection is identified swiftly and contained medically. But sometimes it invades with insidious stealth, either by destroying the heart muscle itself or by narrowing the coronary arteries to the point of no return. I never knew which brand of rejection—muscle or arterial—ruined David's heart; no one in Columbia's transplant program would tell me. Still, it was no secret among gossiping patients that David's heart didn't last as long as it was supposed to; he didn't get anywhere near the time that had been expected for a teenager with a transplant.

How could I be envious of that? A twist of fate and the passage of time showed that I had been the more fortunate one all along. The eight weeks I spent on the waiting list might just have been the lucky break that saved my life and set me up for the miraculously long run of post-transplant years to come. I was not able to avoid the atrophy that settled into my muscles during my long stint of immobility in a hospital bed, but I managed to get an excellent heart—eventually: one that was young, healthy, and so well-suited to the particulars of my body that it seemed to have been mine even before it was placed in my chest. It was a heart worth waiting—and waiting—for.

11

I TURNED TWENTY-FIVE IN THE HOSPITAL.

Scott arrived first thing in the morning with a croissant in hand, an unlit candle stuck in its middle. He stayed with me until evening and then left just as my friend Jill dropped by for a quick birthday hello.

She looked spectacular.

I wondered if Scott had noticed this on his way out. Jill was always an attractive, eye-catching young woman, but tonight she dazzled in a close-fitting blue-and-white polka-dot dress. She was on her way to a party with her boyfriend. Through a sob-stopping lump in my throat, I told her she was a sight for sore eyes: just beautiful.

"And you're looking much better today—with your hair all nice and clean." A few days earlier, Jill had come to visit and I'd asked if she would wash my hair for me in the bathroom sink (I couldn't possibly stand up in the shower). It had been weeks since my Philadelphia shampoo, and my scalp was oily and itching. With Jill's help, I broke my own rule of inactivity and got up out of bed just long enough for a cursory lather and rinse, while hugging the basin for support. I began struggling for air before all the suds were out, and Jill suggested gently that we skip the conditioner. But we both knew that a proper shampoo had also been skipped.

Now she was complimenting me on a ponytail of hair that was, really, only half clean. But thanks to Jill, the itch was somewhat relieved.

Before she left, she handed me a small box with sparkly gift wrap. "Open it when you feel like it," she said. I thanked her, returned her kiss on the cheek with one of my own, and placed the box on my bedside table.

I still hadn't opened it when my father and Beverly arrived an hour later. They came into my hospital room with celebratory clamor, bringing with them a lobster dinner (for one) so that we could mark this milestone birthday together. They'd been toting meals to my bedside almost every night—steak, pasta, Chinese food—often from the best New York restaurants. My lack of appetite didn't deter them; night after night they'd arrive at my door with a shopping bag full of dinner (complete with cloth napkin, silverware, and separate plates for salad and entrée); along with the food, they would serve up some welcome company and light conversation that took the spotlight off my sick heart for a precious few minutes. Then they'd leave my room quickly, off to have their own dinner somewhere else—somewhere without an EKG monitor staring at them. Even on my birthday night, I was the only one digging in to the mountain of food they'd brought along. My father and Beverly stood patiently on either side of my bed and watched over me as I ate, just as they'd done almost every night since my arrival at Columbia. My birthday celebration was no different, with my usual polite showing of a hearty appetite that was, in fact, nonexistent. Crumbs would fall between my bedsheets, just like they always did, and once again I would leave them there, fearing the heart-scary effort it would take for me to clear them away with a vigorous sweep of my hand. Yes, this night was going to be like all the others I'd spent on the waiting list: eating a fine meal without a dining partner and sleeping amid the crumbs.

Except tonight I had lobster.

Two or three bites, anyway.

"Maybe one of the nurses would like to finish these," I said, pointing to the hefty claws that lay untouched on my plate. "Unless one of you wants them."

"No, thanks," my father said. "We're off to Carnegie Hall. Some Wagner tonight. And Brahms, I think. Lovely. You know, the Violin Concerto in D: *da-dee, da-dum, dum dum dum.*" He'd always loved to hum music to me this way, delighting in how easily I could decode his *da-dums*.

"Nice. Sounds like a fun evening for you guys," I said, folding my napkin and placing it on top of a heap of uneaten string beans and hash-brown potatoes.

Beverly tossed the corner of her light cashmere wrap around her shoulder. This was the first signal: my parents were on their way out.

"Happy, happy birthday, darling daughter," my father said, leaning in for a hug.

I lifted my arms up slowly to return the embrace. "Thanks, Dad, for the food; it was great."

Beverly stepped around to the other side of my bed, the thin heels of her evening sandals clicking on the tile floor. She lowered her head to give me a kiss. "Love you. Happy birthday."

"Love you too, both of you," I said, closing my eyes at the touch of Beverly's lips against my forehead. When I opened them again in the next second, tears had already welled up, heavy and obvious. Beverly turned toward the window and brushed away a few of her own, then lightly click-stepped her way back to the door to rejoin my father. As they stood there together, hand in hand, I could see in their tight, forced smiles that there was a part of both of them that didn't want to leave me just yet, especially on my twenty-fifth birthday. But I knew there was another part of them—a stronger part, perhaps—that couldn't wait to step out of my room, out of the ugliness of Columbia-Presbyterian Hospital and into the warm New York City night where fancy lobster dinners didn't come with a side serving of V-fib, and the melodies of Brahms rang through the concert halls.

"It's okay. You can go," I said, my eyes like delicate teacups filled to the brim, ready to spill.

"Pasta marinara tomorrow?" my father asked.

"Sounds good."

I blinked, and the first drops fell from my eyes. Damn it. I wanted to hold them until my parents left. I wanted to be able to take from this birthday visit—and all of my parents' visits—whatever I could that was good, and not ruin it.

There was love worth savoring in the food they brought me. In the nightly visits. In the videos they left at my bedside. In the blanket Beverly knitted for me every day I was in the hospital, sitting at the edge of my bed in the afternoons with balls of white and blue yarn on her lap, needles clacking together softly, constantly. But there were no words. We never talked about the waiting, the V-fib that almost killed me time and again, the imminent loss of my sick heart. My father and Beverly had no wisdom or comfort to pass along when it came to something as strange and as achingly sad as the heart transplant that awaited their twenty-five-year-old daughter. There were no strings they could pull to speed up the waiting process and make a donor heart immediately available, so I pretended not to notice when I saw my father follow a doctor into the hall one day like a puppy dog, trailing after him with the question that no one on the heart transplant team ever liked to hear: "How's she doing on the list?"

"She's still number one," I heard the doctor reply, dry as a bone.

"And that's good. That's the best, right? I mean, what more can we possibly do? Is there anything else we can do?"

The uncharacteristic entreaty in my father's voice twisted me into knots. Oh, my poor, helpless dad.

The doctor cut him off. "We've done everything we can do. Now we just wait."

"Sure. Sure. Okay." My father was forced to retreat. He had no power here. His doctor gods didn't either.

And now my father and Beverly couldn't tolerate the final moments of my birthday visit. Neither could I. Their exit required a bright green light from me, so I told them—again—that they could go. It was okay. Thanks for the birthday dinner. See you tomorrow.

With a quick wave, they were out the door, and I was left alone with the remainder of my tears.

But my nighttime visitations were not over. Soon the evening juice cart would arrive. I looked forward to it. A nurse's aide came around to each patient's room at bedtime, offering up graham crackers and a smile, plus a variety of juices from her cart. I always chose Hawaiian Punch—"The kid stuff again, right?" she'd say—and I sipped it slowly, slurping like a six-year-old, alternating swallows with little bites of sweet cracker. *My first-grade teacher used to give us these same grahams as a snack*, I'd recall, with the arrival of the juice cart night after night. *After we munched at our desks, she'd tell us to put our heads down, close our eyes, and think about something nice—like a party or a day at the beach.* Now, twenty-five years old, in a hospital bed with EKG wires stuck to my chest and shoulders, I reached back in my memory and pulled into the present the sense of calm that used to come over my tiny, sleepy body back in first grade, when I folded my arms on the desk in front of me and laid my head gently down for some happy-time rest. The teacher would walk around the room and place two fingers on each child's shoulder—just for a moment—and it would feel to every comfy-wumfy one of us that we were being tucked in with love.

Now the juice cart was my good-night kiss.

Two graham crackers, a Dixie cupful of Hawaiian Punch, thirty seconds spent studying my heart lines on the EKG monitor—and then nighty-night. Another day of waiting gone by. Maybe my new heart would come tonight, in the middle of the noisy, restless hospital darkness: the wildest, most unbelievable dream-come-true.

Or maybe it would come tomorrow.

Dr. Ganz told me it would come soon. Very soon. He was leaving for a trip to Paris with his wife—a fortieth-birthday celebration—and expected that I would be transplanted while he was away. "I bet you'll have your heart by the time I come back," he said, smiling down at me with his usual kindness. "I'll be gone two weeks."

Two weeks?

"Just think about it. The next time I see you, you'll be out of here." He rolled his eyes to the ceiling, back down, and then wall-to-wall, left to right. "You'll be on the fourth floor just a few days after surgery, walking the halls with your new heart."

I wasn't smiling.

"Why the long face? I think it's going to happen for you, Amy. Soon. I really do. You're number one on the list. You should get a heart any day now. Within two weeks—almost for sure."

There. He'd said it again: two weeks! How was I supposed to survive two weeks with my doctor so far away from me, on a carefree vacation that didn't take my worsening health into consideration at all? Sure, a donor heart might become available over the next two weeks—but would I be alive to accept it? Who would watch over my life while Dr. Ganz was traipsing through Paris?

Who would save me?

The episodes of V-fib were under control now, thanks to a combination of several powerful antiarrhythmia medications and my self-imposed state of inertia. But I still needed expert medical management on a daily basis—fine-tuning that I had entrusted to Dr. Ganz. He'd been doing his best to keep me alive for a month by then, eking out the last bits of function from my sick heart, and I needed him to continue—especially now, since there were new signs that my heart muscle was getting even weaker. A most overwhelming fatigue had begun to set into my body, heavier and more limiting as the hours passed, and each day I found that I had less energy to do the simple things I'd done the day before: put on lipstick in anticipation of Scott's early morning arrival, or brush my teeth in bed and spit into the little pan that lay on my lap. And one morning, when a nurse handed me the usual damp washcloth ("for your privates") and left the room, as always, long enough for me to wipe between my legs, I realized that over the previous twenty-four hours, I'd somehow lost the strength to clean myself. When the nurse returned with a fresh pair of underpants, I told her not to bother. I wasn't up for a change today.

I didn't need another rattling episode of V-fib to remind me how quickly I was dying and how unstoppably. Clean underwear was enough.

"But two weeks!" I said, objecting to my doctor's Paris vacation in a way he wouldn't understand. "Dr. Ganz, really!"

"Yes, just two, isn't that great? A new heart while I'm away," he said.

All through his optimistic ramblings, one plea continued to screech through my mind: *Don't leave me!*

I had been left every day since arriving at Columbia. That's what happens to sick people who must remain tethered to their hospital beds for an extended period of time: they get left. It's unavoidable. Every visitor who comes will go. Every on-duty nurse will eventually be off duty. And every doctor who steps into your hospital room will soon walk out again. Some doctors will disappear for two weeks at a time, and when they go this way they leave you scared out of your mind.

The thought of Dr. Ganz's absence devastated me. I cried and cried after he left my room, until my heartbeat clued into my emotions and began to thump ominously. I reached for another tissue and allowed myself one final whimper before heeding the familiar danger call that was coming from my sick heart. This cry had to stop—now.

I was gathering together the mound of crumpled tissues that lay across my chest when the transplant psychiatrist, Dr. Stein, walked in. Oh, no, he finally had me in his clutches, caught teary-eyed in the middle of a meltdown. And, as usual, I was not in the mood to talk.

Not to him, anyway.

Dr. Stein was part of the transplant team, which included a dedicated cadre of cardiologists, surgeons, nurses, physical therapists, social workers, nutritionists, and even dentists. I didn't choose Dr. Stein; he was assigned to me, as he was to all pre-transplant patients, who he would evaluate psychologically as part of their wait-list requirements. Since I had remained in the hospital after being placed on the transplant list, Dr. Stein had made it his business to stand at the foot of my bed every few days and try to strike up some conversation. From time to time, I'd oblige him with a few paltry shavings of my thoughts and feelings, but most often I gave him only mumblings of obvious complaint ("When will I get a heart already?") and so avoided being fodder for his brand of bedside psychotherapy. I found his visits to be a nuisance more than anything else, and as the days passed I would come to feel more and more sorry for the guy, with his stiff, awkward body language and the way he pulled at his sparse smattering of chin hair during the long silences that hung in the tense space between us. Our talks had terrible starts and stops, gaping holes, and uncomfortable final moments, wherein one of us would get up the courage to wrap up our empty exchange for the day and say something like, "Okay, then. All right. Okay. We're done? Yes? Done? See you, then. Good? Good."

And through this staccato of words we would agree: our discussion had come to its usual sticky end.

But when Dr. Stein arrived at my door today, on the heels of the Paris-bound Dr. Ganz, he sensed he just might have hit the jackpot. Something was up, something that might lead me to engage in a real discussion with him for once.

In spite of myself, I helped him out.

"Dr. Ganz is leaving me—for two weeks," I told him.

I'd opened the window wider than ever. Dr. Stein flew right in with a couple of suggestions I might want to consider. I probably had a lot of "feelings" about people coming and going, visiting me and then returning to their healthy lives, while I had no choice but to remain in the hospital—indefinitely. He told me this was understandable and then laid on the emphasis by using himself as an example. "I can see how it happens. Like, for instance, I'm going away for an extended weekend in the Hamptons tomorrow. I'll be relaxing at the beach for three days, and then when I come back I'll be tanned and rested. And you'll probably still be in this room. It's got to make you feel angry, really angry. I think I would feel a whole lot of anger if I were in your place."

Anger?

There was some anger inside me. But it was buried beneath layers and layers of a much more urgent emotion that demanded my full attention every moment: raw, all-encompassing fear. No one recognized that feeling, not Dr. Ganz and not even this transplant psychiatrist. They didn't appreciate the extent to which I was caught up in being afraid of my own body. Hell, I could hardly indulge in the luxury of anger. I was too busy trying to help save my life—clinging to the people and things I believed were saving it along with me. Like Dr. Ganz, arrhythmia expert and most kindly soul. Like Fred, the nurse who knew just what to do when the alarm sounded above my door. And like my hospital room, where I relied on the safety of the heartbeat monitor that watched over me 24/7. Give Dr. Ganz leave for a long vacation or send Fred home for a three-day break—or wheel me out of my room on a stretcher, down three floors to have an echocardiogram—and I was overwhelmed by the most intense fear.

I could have fleshed out a few of these scenarios for Dr. Stein, or given him examples of recent experiences that showed fear reigning supreme over anger. I considered sharing with him what had happened to me several days earlier as I lay on a stretcher in an unfamiliar hallway, unattended and alone, waiting to have a diagnostic test that would complete the last step in placing me on the transplant list: how I'd spun into a vortex of fear and thought I might die right then and there—and this was not an exaggeration of possibility. No one was monitoring my heart. There was no alarm attached to me that would alert anyone if I went into V-fib. For the first time in weeks, I was without the safety of wires and a nearby defibrillator cart. My heart would either break into a lethal arrhythmia in that hallway or it wouldn't, and no one seemed to care or even notice. How maddening, right? It was enough to make any patient angry—stranded on a stretcher in that deserted hallway, ten minutes passing, then twenty, then thirty—but all I felt was paralyzing fear. Placing two fingers against the pulse in my neck, I counted my own heartbeats, monitoring the rhythm so I might scream for help if I felt too many wild skips in a row. I focused only on keeping myself alive until a doctor or skilled nurse arrived to take that responsibility back from me. It was an hour and a half before the journey came to an end and someone from the transport staff wheeled me back to my hospital room. When I arrived there, safe but hardly sound, I didn't breathe angry fire, only a shuddering exhalation of relief. I was no longer left alone to die, and I could finally stop counting heartbeats.

I decided to keep this story to myself and not share anything more with Dr. Stein than I had to. I told him simply that I wasn't feeling very much anger.

He widened his eyes like a doll, not believing me. "It would be only normal."

"I said I'm not angry!" At least not until that moment.

Dr. Stein lifted his hands up by his shoulders like an accused criminal showing he's got nothing to hide, "Look, I'm only suggesting something here . . . based on what I observe."

"What you observe? I barely speak to you. You just assume I'm supposed to fit into a sick-person model you read about in Psych 101 or 102 maybe. But I can tell you, when you try to push this anger thing on me it just makes you look like a big idiot—standing in your ivory tower, telling me what I feel. Don't kid yourself. You don't know the first thing about me, *Doctor.*"

These were more words than this guy had gotten out of me in three weeks. He pulled slowly at his goatee in silence, his eyes glazing over, half focused on my face.

I jumped in with a thought I'd been keeping under wraps for weeks. "And you can't even look me in the eye!"

"I have a wandering eye," he said.

And left.

12

I BROUGHT THE ENDS OF MY LONG HAIR FORWARD AND INSPECTED the profuse matting that had set in. It didn't look much like mine anymore; strands had turned to clumps, just as I knew they would. Not even Beverly knew how to navigate a comb through my unruly curls, and I didn't have enough strength to untangle them myself. I'd been lying down in a hospital bed for about four weeks now, and most of what I could see of myself (without getting out of bed to look in the bathroom mirror) had become unrecognizable due to neglect and illness. Dry cracked nails, swollen ankles like overstuffed sausages, bluish veins running beneath pale tissue-thin skin. Flesh-and-bone arms poking through the hospital gown like two angular twigs.

I thought to myself, *I'm ugly*.

Scott would not agree, I knew. It was almost 8 A.M. and soon he would arrive and tell me—again—that I was beautiful. He managed to say this every morning and appear completely earnest. Sometimes I even believed him, but then overnight, in his absence, I'd look down at my wasted body and arrive at a different conclusion. I was sick; sick was ugly; I was ugly.

"Hello, beautiful girl." Scott paused beneath the doorframe. He smiled wide and true, eyes lighting up just at the sight of me.

I tried to sit up a little more and look prettier for him.

"I brought you some breakfast." He lifted a brown paper bag to prove it. "Carrot muffin."

As his arm reached out to the side, bag in hand, an aura of fluorescence came up behind him, a reflection off the white tiled hallway. And there he was again, just like every morning of my hospital stay, strikingly framed in light and appearing almost imaginary: my angel.

Scott.

He placed the brown paper bag on the table beside my bed. As I reached for my breakfast muffin, he took one final sip of coffee from a deli travel cup and tossed it into the wastebasket at the other end of the room. I watched the graceful arc of white Styrofoam up through the air, and then followed its on-target descent—plunk—into the empty pail. When I turned my head back to look at Scott, he wasn't there.

"Down here," he said.

He was kneeling at my bedside.

"What are you doing down there, silly?" I eased my torso over to the side of the bed and found him below, arm extended toward me.

"Oh, Scotty!"

There was a small blue velvet box in his hand. He pried it open.

"Amy—my love." He paused, eyes gleaming. "I was wondering—will you marry me?"

Scott was already on his way up from his knees when I shouted out, "Yes!"

He slid the pear-shaped diamond ring onto my finger.

"Yes! I will marry you, my sweet, sweet love!"

Uh-oh.

Too much excitement for a dangerously sick body.

I felt my heart begin its arrhythmic dance. Instinct caused my arm to swing up and across my chest in a protective motion, "I can't scream like that, Scotty. My heart—"

"It's okay. I know."

"But you've made me so happy. I want to jump right out of this bed, but I can't. . . ."

"Don't worry. You don't have to move. Let me move," he said, climbing up one leg at a time and stretching out alongside me. Nose to nose in a hospital bed, we kissed and smiled, smiled and kissed, just like any young newly engaged couple might. And my heart calmed down. For the moment.

Then it hit me again: I'd just gotten engaged—and it was a surprise. Scott and I had never spoken about marriage in a concrete way. A few high-pitched squeaks escaped my lips. "*Eee! Eee! Eee!*"

Scott sat up in bed and laughed out loud, smiling like his old self—ear to ear—with that genuine warmth and sparkle that endeared him to almost everyone he met. How beautiful he was! Look at this handsome, loving man beside me. He was the finest person I had ever known. And I was going to marry him.

Again it was time to steady my heart—damn it—before the alarm went off above my door. I knew I'd been cutting it too close. I simply could not allow this kind of thrill to run through my body; pure unfettered joy was a dangerous risk. I took a slow deep breath and let it out. "I love you, Scotty. But I have to be very quiet right now."

Scott lay back down beside me, nose to nose once again, our heads sharing the small hospital pillow. He wrapped his arms around me and gave my poor heart the rest it needed. I wasn't able to return his embrace with the energy it deserved, but he understood why.

Our happiness could never be easy. But it could be enough.

There was joy in the days following our engagement to prop me up with renewed energy. I asked my nurse to bring me paper and pen, and I'd fill the hours scribbling my new name over and over again, in script and then in print. Beverly showed up with an array of brides' magazines, and together we tore out photo after photo of gowns we both liked. My hospital room was decorated with an array of dress options hastily affixed to the walls with medical tape; my nurses cast votes for the prettiest one. Dr. Ganz, back from Paris, liked the classic high-neck one in antique white.

Enchantment was unmistakably in the air.

There was a dreamlike quality to my engagement. Long after Scott and I were married, the image of him dropping to his knees beside my bed would appear to me like a dream—not so much for its sense of being too good to be true as for the way the story line moved forward without anyone's questioning whether it was nonsensical. In dreams we can do the fantastic: ride a bicycle that has wings for tires; row a boat through a lake of lions; soar above the limitations of severe illness. It was the surreal quality of Scott's proposal that allowed *yes* to flow from my lips, carrying us both along in reverie and holding off the massive elephant that must have been pounding at the door.

There was a distinct possibility that an attack of arrhythmia would kill me before a donor heart became available, that I'd be buried with an engagement ring on my finger that never had the chance to glitter beyond the walls of my hospital room, and that I would not live to see my wedding day. But Scott endeavored in all earnestness to marry me; he asked my father for my hand, secretly enlisted the help of his mother and Beverly in picking out a ring, and conjured up words for a proposal befitting the woman he loved. Never once, before or after our marriage, would Scott let on that he had experienced any trepidation when asking me to marry him. I would survive the waiting period, and we would live together for many, many years after my surgery—without a doubt.

The doctors had told us that a heart transplant—whenever I was lucky enough to get it—would not be a cure; it would just be the substitution of one serious health problem for another, a permanent state of immunosuppression for heart failure. But for Scott this was a more than adequate trade-off. Transplant would allow me to live. It would allow him to place a second ring on my finger—a wedding band—and this was all that mattered. Scott moved forward, intent on marrying me.

My father plowed ahead as well, wrapped up in his own dream. No sooner had I said yes to Scott's proposal than my father and Beverly had booked a place for our wedding. I overheard my dad asking a doctor, "After her transplant, how long should we wait to have the wedding?" The answer was that it could take one year post-transplant for me to recover and be ready for marriage. This was all that my father needed to hear.

Even though there was no date from which he could count off 365 days of recovery time (he would have to begin counting from a transplant date that did not yet exist), my father assumed that June twenty-fourth of the following year would work just fine. He put a deposit down at the Pierre Hotel in New York City—not just hundreds but thousands of nonrefundable dollars. Only recently, my father had dropped to his own knees beside me, begging me to fight for my life; now Scott had taken his turn in kneeling by my bedside, proposing a marriage that would ensure that my life would go on. It must go on—I was going to be married at the Pierre! Beverly began contemplating color schemes for tablecloths and napkins.

Elephant, be gone.

We all played our parts in the dream that was my engagement. Everyone who entered my room seemed to have a hand in keeping the reverie going. But for me, living with a heart as sick as mine meant that even the most wonderful dream would have to be part nightmare.

Just two weeks after my engagement, I woke up in the morning, looked at the gray-green hospital walls surrounding me, and decided I'd had enough of waiting for a new heart. The days seemed endless and futile. The many nights I'd spent watching the local news, guiltily hoping to see a car accident—or, better still, a multivehicle pileup that would yield a couple of brain-dead organ donors—had taken their toll, making the gleam of my engagement ring irrelevant. A nurse came in with my 7 A.M. pre-medicine buttered toast that was supposed to ease the intense nausea that followed my morning pills, but I knew it would not help at all. I nibbled at the crust a bit and then put the plate aside. Why bother eating? It was the beginning of another day in a hospital bed, tolerating visits from a string of doctors, a painful IV change (hardly any fresh veins left), a degrading sponge bath, and a line of motionless hours passed in lonely silence—waiting for a goddamn heart. And to make it all worse, Scott wasn't coming this morning; he'd finally given in to my incessant prodding for him to take a day off from the hospital. I had only myself to blame.

I reached for the toast again and took a bite. Yesterday, I'd eaten two pieces just like it, and they'd tasted just fine. Today, this one tasted like hospital. I spit it into my hand.

The phone rang, and it was Valerie, calling from our dorm room. She hadn't come to visit me over the past few weeks; there were final exams to tackle and then the start of her summer job at a law firm. But she checked in as often as I could abide; talking on the phone exhausted me.

It was only because Valerie's phone call was the first of the morning that she would also be the first person to hear me say, my voice quivering and precariously breathy, "I've had enough. I can't sit in this body or in this stupid hospital bed one more second. I have to get out of here—now."

There was a window I could open, I told her. I could ask my nurse to make me some more toast or something, pull out my IV while she was away on the trumped-up errand, and climb out the window of my room.

"Amy, you can't do that. You wouldn't."

Oh, yes, I would.

The young woman who had pleaded with the doctors, "Save me! I love my Scotty!" no longer wished to be saved. The saving was killing her.

Within minutes of hanging up with a tearful Valerie, Dr. Stein arrived. (I would learn after my transplant that Valerie had contacted him, calling the transplant department after we got off the phone and asking to speak to the staff psychiatrist. She told him I sounded like I might do something crazy.) Now it was Dr. Stein's turn to save me, not with a shock to the chest and a flood of antiarrhythmia chemicals but with talk, the same brand I'd found so useless over the past few weeks.

This was not a routine visit. Regular drop bys from Dr. Stein had practically ceased with his telling me that I should just call if I wanted to talk. Fat chance. Today he moved in closer than ever to my bedside, dropped his jaw open like a marionette, and stood there breathing through his mouth for a few seconds while conjuring up what he hoped would be a therapeutically useful opening line: "I hear you're feeling . . . distressed today."

Brilliant.

"Yes. I don't want to do this anymore. I need to have some peace—which means I have to get out of this hospital room. And maybe even out of this body." I spoke calmly and without emotion, deliberately self-possessed.

"I see."

"No, you don't. And don't try to give me any psycho medications. I am not crazy. I am just done."

"All right. But will you just try something with me first? It's a sort of mind exercise. I think it will help you relax and feel less anxious."

"Wrong again. I'm not feeling anxious. I'm feeling determined. I'm not sitting in this bed dying anymore." He looked down at the ground and squeezed his lips tight together as if suddenly tasting lemons. I could see the circle of scalp peeking through his thinning hair, and when he lifted his head back up and looked right at me, I noticed his wandering eye bouncing around in its socket. Seemed to me like this doctor could use some saving himself.

I agreed to let him lead me through the relaxation exercise.

"Great. Close your eyes."

Dr. Stein told me to breathe slow and deep. Then there was some counting backward to keep my mind busy; I was supposed to picture myself on a ladder or something, stepping down rungs. Breathing. Counting. Descending. This went on for a while and then finally, as a test of my newly calmed state, Dr. Stein lifted my arm a few inches off the bed and let go. Only after I stopped the fall did I realize what had been intended by this trial: my arm was supposed to have gone limp. I was supposed to be relaxed, but I wasn't. Dr. Stein and I both sensed this, and I wasn't sure who felt worse about it.

"I think I'm feeling better now. Thanks," I said. In other words, *Get out of my room and leave me alone.*

"Good. That's good," he said. "I'll check back with you later, if that's okay?"

I threw him a bone. "Sure."

But I did not see Dr. Stein later. Before enough hours would pass to bring him back to my hospital room for another round of mind exercises, a young resident doctor rushed into my room without knocking. "We've got a heart for you. Stop eating now!" he said, and was gone as quickly as he came. I looked down at the outline of my legs beneath the white hospital blanket and realized that I'd brought them toward my chest, pulling myself up into a full sitting position, unsupported by pillows for the first time in over a month.

Scott was summoned from his one day, of respite from the hospital. He was at his mother's house for the day, feeling the whole time that he never should have left me alone. It was about an hour's drive to Columbia; he and his stepfather left immediately.

The traffic was terrible, Scott would tell me in later years, so he jumped out of the car and sprinted up Broadway, leaving his stepfather to drive the remaining thirty blocks to the hospital. He would describe it as the most unnerving, frustrating experience of his life: trying desperately to get to a destination, a precious life hanging in the balance—and bumper-to-bumper traffic on upper Broadway. A nightmare, he said. Scott was propelled forward by the thought of my needing him and his not being there.

He blew into my room. There were no words, only a dive onto my bed. Scott held on to me, steady and strong. As always, I was quickly comforted by the safety of his embrace, but at this moment his protection scared me as well: how was I going to let go of this man and allow myself to be wheeled into an operating room where they would take my heart out?

I began to scream, full and forceful, paying no regard to my racing heart. My high-pitched wail grew louder with each repetition: *Aaahhh! Aaahhh!* Each shriek fed off the strength of the preceding one, building in intensity and hysteria until I had spiraled completely out of control. "They're going to cut my heart out! I'm going to die on the operating table! They're going to kill me!" Scott didn't even try to respond, he just held my shaking body for what seemed like a very long time. "I'm going to die! I'm going to die!"

A nurse arrived with a sedative injection.

I didn't have much experience with sedation, except for the forgetting medicine that had arrived along with the defibrillator paddles (when I was lucky), and some light anesthesia for a tooth extraction when I was a child. I imagined that the injection would render me entirely complacent, accepting of everything and anything, which is a dangerous state of being for any hospital patient. Sedation, I feared, was sure to take the fight out of me: the will and determination that had kept me alive long enough to get the heart that was going to be transplanted into me this very day. Once I let go and allowed my mind to detach from the business of keeping me alive, I would put my body and brain completely and helplessly into the hands of the doctors in the operating room—none of whom I knew well or had reason to trust.

Doing what was best for my sick heart, I knew at that moment, would mean surrendering my better judgment. But I would do it. I needed to succomb in order to be saved.

Two hours later, my stretcher rolled down the hall and past a line of people: Scott and his mother, brother, and stepfather, Beverly, and Fred, my nurse. And then, finally, there was my father, who raised his hand, waved as my stretcher slid past him, and called out, "See you in a few hours!"

I was pretty sure I'd never see any of them again.

A new heart was transplanted into my body on June 24, 1988. Exactly one year later, Scott and I were married at the Pierre Hotel on the very date that had been chosen by my father back when I was still waiting on the transplant list without a new heart in sight. Perhaps my dad had a knack for picking dates. Or maybe fate was playing out its hand stealthily, giving the appearance of simple coincidence. But whatever the force behind the momentous reappearance of June 24, the effect was mystical—enough to raise the hair on your arms if you let it.

Maybe true love can work magic after all.

13

FOR THE PEOPLE WHO SAT IN THE WAITING ROOM THE NIGHT OF MY heart transplant, the end of the surgery would also signal the end of my illness; that was how they understood it. When my father waved a casual *so long* as my stretcher slipped behind the closing doors of an elevator, he expected me to return to him later that night as a daughter who had been cured. There would be cause for celebration once all that cutting and sewing was over and done with. The sick heart would have been removed. Gone. A thing of the past.

But meanwhile there was tension. My father, Beverly, Scott, and Scott's parents and brother sat knee to knee on the threadbare couches that were the only alternative to pacing the deserted hospital corridors at midnight, and then at one in the morning, and then again at two. By 3 A.M., nervous hunger had begun to stir in at least one of the knotted stomachs in the crowd.

My father sought to rally the troops behind the call of his implacable sweet tooth. "I do believe I saw an all-night Dunkin' Donuts on my way in here, did I not?" He canvassed the waiting-room assemblage for a volunteer. "Anyone up for a quick doughnut run?"

"I'll go," Scott's brother said.

Offer accepted.

"Why don't you get a dozen or so," my father suggested, having removed himself from the active part of the mission. "Chocolate ones. Chocolate frosted, chocolate in the middle, on the side, dipped, sprinkled, glazed—"

"I got it. You want chocolate."

"Yup. Anyone else have a request?"

No one did. The weary contingent would be content to pick from among my father's chocolate choices.

Scott's brother set out alone on the mission, braving the deserted streets of Washington Heights so he might calm my father's anxiety with fried dough and chocolate. He returned to the waiting room within minutes—task accomplished—carrying in the crook of his arm a cardboard box containing a full baker's dozen: twelve of the chocolate variety plus one sugar-powdered jelly-filled doughnut, an oddball he'd tossed in just for the hell of it.

My father was the first at the box.

"Ah, yes, delicious!" he said, fluttering his fingers in that Groucho Marx way while eyeballing the array of doughnuts as he made his final selection. "I'll take this one. Perfect!"

He reached his hand down into the crowd of chocolate options and pulled out the lone jelly doughnut. It was the first and last one that he ate. The twelve chocolate doughnuts remained in the box, nestled between sheets of waxy paper, untouched.

That was the story I was told; waiting-room anecdotes would come to me in bits and pieces with increasing frequency (and perhaps inventiveness) as the post-surgery years unfolded. The tale of the late-night doughnut run was an entirely believable one. But there were many others that seemed less plausible once they made it to my ears. Beverly had one of these to tell—a story she recounted to me in some detail many years later—that had the distinctive ring of imaginary hindsight. When I pressed her on it, she would retract just the slightest bit, and only temporarily; how could she have remembered such a jarring occurrence if it had never happened? Her surgery-night story was not the sort of thing a person could ever forget, and it was certainly not the kind that someone would make up. It was more like what might be encountered in a nightmare.

But Beverly said it happened. Or probably happened. "I tell you, I remember him walking in with it—bringing it over to us, I think, in a little metal tin," she told me, for the second time.

Following the lead of her words, I would use my imagination to complete the picture in my mind: it had been a kidney-shaped metallic bowl, the kind that is often found sitting on top of a supply chest in a doctor's office, with cotton balls in it or a pair of tongs.

"Your surgeon, Doctor Solomon, came in after the operation, and he showed it to us—your heart. It was just lying there—all flat—like a piece of liver at the butcher shop. He said something like, 'Can you believe she had this thing inside of her? It's a wonder she's alive.'"

The rounded contours of my heart had been, in fact, completely replaced by limp flaccidness, all of the heart's muscle having been obliterated by disease. Other sources besides Beverly —reliable doctors whose recollections carried more weight —told me my heart had been a "total pancake" and that the communal sense in the operating room was that the extent of my cardiomyopathy was even worse than any of the pre-transplant diagnostic tests had indicated. Pancakes like this one didn't keep patients alive very long. The doctors were stunned that I hadn't died; it had been that bad a pump.

Mine was a sick heart for the record books.

But had it really been spectacle enough to prompt a judicious level-headed surgeon to whisk the bloody thing out of the operating room in its entirety, carry it down the hall, and show it off to a waiting room full of people who could not stomach a few bites of doughnut?

Unlikely.

"There's no way, Bev. I can't imagine that Dr. Solomon would bring my heart to you in a bowl. Dad would have passed out on the spot."

"I know it sounds strange. But I tell you, I remember seeing it. The doctor made a big deal about how flat it was—pointing to it and explaining."

"Maybe it's the *pancake* word you're remembering, and the rest is just imagination. He probably came in and told you how my heart had looked to him—back in the operating room. Doctors don't show hearts to families. Not everyone wants to see something like that."

"I don't know. It wasn't too bad to look at, really."

"My dead heart—all detached and everything—in a bowl, for God's sake?"

"Well, maybe you're right. Maybe he didn't show it to us. I'm not so sure about it, I guess. Gosh, though, I swear I remember seeing it."

Scott later told me that he was one hundred percent sure that he, for one, hadn't seen my heart that night. "I would have lost it," he said.

Scott's mother told me the same thing when I asked her: No, the surgeon had not shown them my heart, thank goodness. What she remembered most vividly was Dr. Solomon coming into the waiting room after having completed his work and telling them how lucky I had been to have survived the many weeks on the waiting list with a flaccid, nearly lifeless pancake for a heart.

"We saved her just in time," he'd said to the roomful of people who so wanted to believe that I had indeed been saved.

But isn't that how it always is? All transplant operations seem to come just in the nick of time. Every heart transplant patient needs to be saved. I was no different. The circumstances of my surgery were hardly out of the ordinary. And Dr. Carl Solomon—the hotshot young cardiac transplant surgeon who'd just finished saving me—had merely carried out his job once again.

There he'd stood, hour after hour beside my anesthetized body, with his perfect hands buried and busy within my chest cavity. He removed the heart that was killing me and replaced it deftly with one that would save me—just like he'd done for another dying patient two weeks earlier, and for another sinking heart-failure victim one week before that.

"Don't let me die," I'd said to him, just a few hours before my surgery. That was all there had been time for. It was clear that Dr. Solomon was in a big rush. He breezed into my hospital room just moments before a stretcher would carry me out of it, and I laid eyes on him for the very first time. His tightly locked jaw told me not to get started with any questions or getting-to-know-you banter; he wasn't talking. He was only maintaining a stationary pose beside my bed for a short moment as a witness to anything I might say, but acting as neither receiver nor responder. Dr. Solomon was only a presence—a handsome man, I noticed—who stood in my direct line of vision as if on display, a hands-off showing of the surgeon who would soon cut out my heart. And I was supposed to lie there in bed and revere him—or something.

"Please, don't let me die," I said again, trying to catch at least one of the blue eyes that had shifted sharply toward the door.

"Right," he said, and was gone.

Dr. Solomon was well used to not letting people die. He knew that by the end of this surgery (which would conclude in the early morning hours) he would have performed "just another everyday miracle," these being the words used by other cardiac transplant surgeons after having used their most select skills in the operating room. There seemed to be something matter-of-fact about the surgical procedure Dr. Solomon was about to carry out, and at the same time it was work that was always breathtaking. Heart transplantation was part of his job as a cardiac surgeon, but it was also, somehow, beyond it; not only would he use his hands to restore life to this young woman, he would use the life of a deceased teenager to do it. Life to death. Death to life. Even a no-frills, silent John Wayne type like Carl Solomon could get caught up in the sheer miracle of it all.

In the span of a single operation, Dr. Solomon got the chance not simply to touch or prod but actually to hold in his hand not one but two hearts: one dying and one lifesaving. And while all surgeons may view themselves as holding life in their hands at one time or another, heart-transplant surgeons have an even greater sense of this phenomenon: they must take hold of a motionless donor heart, place it into the cavity where the transplant recipient's heart had once been, make all necessary surgical reattachments with careful precision, and then take the final leap of faith that will tell whether the evening of brilliant surgical toil has been successful. They must remove the patient from the life force of the heart-lung machine and see if the new heart beats on its own.

Sometimes it does.

Sometimes it does not.

Dr. Solomon was pleased to report to the waiting-room group that the donated heart had burst into robust, vigorous beats from the moment the heart-lung machine had been switched off. My new heart just flew on its own, needing no prodding or artificial stimulation to get going. This was a very good sign. The next forty-eight hours would be critical, though; they would show whether the heavy doses of immunosuppressive medications now flooding my bloodstream were enough to hold off a dangerous episode of rejection. Transplant surgery was only the first step; it was the carefully controlled inhibition of my immune system that would keep me alive through this night and, if I was lucky, for years to come. And at no point in my transplant life could I stop taking these medicines, since it was only their suppressive powers that could prevent my body from laying siege to a heart that would forever be, in essence, foreign.

Dr. Solomon had given my parents their first basic lesson in heart-transplant survival: sustained immunosuppression. "She's well medicated now and doing fine," he told them. It would be a good idea to go home now and get some rest; I was likely to sleep for the next day, at least.

But Scott, Beverly, and my father wanted to see me before leaving that night. They stood in the hallway of the post-surgical ICU until my anesthetized body was wheeled past them on a stretcher.

"You weren't easy to look at," my father would tell me in later years, "There wasn't a place on you that didn't have some kind of pipe coming out of it. And you were just the loveliest shade of gray. Like the Bride of Frankenstein."

For years to come, Scott would remind me that I'd had "something gigantic" sticking out of my abdomen for the first couple of days after my surgery and that to look at it made him recoil with queasiness."

"You were a mess," he'd tell me, without apology.

And I would always imagine the post-surgery hideousness of me and how much love must have been shielding Scott's eyes from it as he sat on the edge of my bed—right beside the very tube that wrenched his guts—when I opened my eyes for the first time since my surgery. He flew to my bedside the moment he saw my eyelashes begin to flutter; he knew it was time to fulfill a promise.

"I'm here, honey, can you see me?"

"Um . . . kind of." Nurse Vera had smeared my eyes with a super-moisturizing swipe of Vaseline.

"I have your ring, remember?"

"Mmm." Words were an effort through the lingering anesthesia.

"The nurse made you take it off before the operation. So now I want to ask you again, because you've had a 'change of heart'—right? Remember how we talked about that?" Scott held his hands out toward me in an offering of something that he hoped I would be alert enough to expect from him at this moment. Soon after our engagement, I'd made him promise to propose to me again after my surgery because I would have a new heart—perhaps one with different love in it. He'd laughed about it at the time, though I warned him in half seriousness that I really meant it; he'd better get on his knees again and give my new heart a chance to say yes.

But knees were out of the question today; the standard ICU bed was just too high for Scott to reach me. So he sat on a sliver of mattress just beside my hip bone, knelt, if only in spirit, and asked if I would love him forever—again.

"Amy, will you marry me?"

"*Whoop!*" A sudden cheer rang out from the nurses' station. Wild applause and hoots of exhilaration came pouring through the speakers built into the ceiling of my room. The sight and sound of Scott's proposal had been recorded and transmitted live to the nurses' station through a video camera positioned just over my bed. Scott had no idea that he was being watched this way, and the surprise startled him at first. Then he laughed and laughed, his spirits lifted by the unexpected crescendo of revelry coming from somewhere down the hall. The sound of our reengagement was confirmation, for anyone who was lucky enough to hear it, that the pure joy of love could be truly infectious—even in the post-surgery cardiac ICU.

I managed to breathe out a contented *yes* before my heavy eyelids gave way again. Someone was lifting my hand, ever so gently. I had a sense of something sliding along the length of my finger, up and up, until it came to a stop. And then I heard another one of those shouts—*Whoop!*—coming from somewhere in the distance.

This second jubilant cry from the nurses' station was the last thing I would remember hearing before drifting back into sweet sleep. Scott had slipped the engagement ring on my finger for the second and last time. He kissed my forehead and floated back to his chair at the far end of the room, elated.

"I feel better. . . ."

I awoke after my transplant for the second time and spoke aloud, with more awareness and clarity than the day before. Someone was there to hear me, I knew; through newly applied layers of

Vaseline, I could make out the blurry outline of Scott's figure slumped in a chair at the far end of my room.

It had been a long, sleepless, white-knuckle night for him, followed by a frustrating day of anticipation; I hadn't regained consciousness—even for a moment—since his second proposal. And now time had spilled over into the late afternoon, with him still watching over me in nervous anticipation. Some forty hours had passed since the surgery that had begun with the grainy whir of a chain saw cutting open the pristine chest of his twenty-five-year-old bride-to-be. My limp body lay before him now in post-surgery inertia, bare-chested, with a thick swath of blood-tinged gauze running down the length of my sternum, hiding the raw newly stitched skin. Just beneath this indelible surgical line lay the wires that would be with me for the rest of my life—bow-tie-style, like the knotted loops at the top of a sneaker, each bow stacked an inch above the one beneath it—pulling the severed edges of my rib cage back together again and holding them there. All this gruesomeness a confirmation of a single, glorious fact: I had received my gift of life.

Indeed.

". . . But I don't know if I want to throw up or go back to sleep." I said.

A gentle swell of laughter rose up from all four corners of the room, the sound of eager if tentative relief. Now I knew for sure that other people were there with me besides Scott.

"Sleep, Amy . . . Amy . . . mee . . . mee. . . ." they suggested in distorted unison, a Greek chorus of sorts, warped by the haze of lingering anesthesia. "Go ahead and let yourself rest . . . est . . . est. We'll be here when you wake up . . . up . . . up. . . ."

"Yeah, even if you're throwing up, we'll be here! You can count on it."

My father was in the room—unmistakably. His words reached me with no echo effect. Still, the heavy pull of sedation did its best to draw me away from the sound of his voice. As I floated in a cloud of semiawareness, the familiar hum of my father's humor remained suspended somewhere between me and the ceiling. I left it hanging there, willingly. I was content to give myself over once again to the seductive, sweet darkness of drug-induced sleep. But as I began to slip away from the lighthearted post-surgery welcome, something grabbed me from the inside out, taking hold of my fading consciousness and shaking it back to life; something vital insisted on my full attention. I knew at once what it was: a sensation right there in my chest, seemingly new to me and at the same time oddly familiar, as if I'd experienced it in a dream once and then lost my sense of it forever. The feeling tugged at my attention and teased it in a way that wrested from my sleepy mind the most impossibly urgent curiosity. I snapped my eyes open in an instant and directed inward every bit of focus I could manage, paying close attention to whatever it was in my body that was beckoning me to connect with it, recognize it for what it was, and give it a name.

Its name was peace.

This was the sensation that had been the silent force behind the words I'd mumbled without forethought as I regained consciousness: "I feel better."

In place of the sick, struggling thud that had lumbered beneath my breastbone, now there was an entirely different feeling: a calm unremarkable pulsing. All at once I remembered that, for most people, heartbeats are barely noticeable.

It was like that for me—once. Yes, I remembered it then: a pulse that doesn't threaten. A heart that doesn't spin out of control. Good health. Effortless health. The health I'd once known.

This small memory of wellness was sufficient enticement for me to continue battling against sleep—if only for another thirty seconds—just to experience feeling myself this way again. I closed my eyes and took one last moment to immerse myself in the most basic joy of simply being all right.

Peace. It was what I'd left behind—strewn along the streets of Philadelphia or seated as a shadow of memory in the third row of a law-school lecture hall. And now, for a brief moment at least, I thought maybe I'd found it again, reclaimed the serenity that had once been mine. A slow smile came to my lips as I gave myself over to the most enticing sedative of all: the promise of a calm heart and an untroubled sleep.

I had been through so much to get here. A disturbing sense of this was still with me in a hazy flash of memory: my last moment of consciousness in the operating room. I'd given myself over to an entirely different kind of slumber back there, a dreadful one, the anticipation of which had caused my features to contort into a rigid grimace: bulging eyes of fear and a gaping mouth that howled a silent scream. Within seconds, an unfamiliar hand had come down at me, plunging hastily from above my face and forcing my breathing into the confines of an oxygen mask without warning or comfort that might ready me or steady me before impact. I was going under, like it or not. The operating-room nurse had already tied my arms down (couldn't she have waited until I was asleep to do that?), having stretched them flat along the length of two slender boards that stuck out at right angles on either side of my body. I darted my eyes quickly from arm to arm (I was trapped!) and then up to the ceiling, toward the faces that peered down from a circle in the sky, high above the operating table: an oval of stadium-style seating set back behind protective glass. Spectators were in the process of finding their seats, smoothing their white coats and settling down for the next few hours, as if they'd just taken their seats in the mezzanine of a Broadway theater.

Everyone can see my breasts, I thought, thoroughly embarrassed, aware that my chest was exposed and that a telltale antiseptic orange-brown stripe of Betadine now ran the length of my torso—neck to navel—along the line of my cleavage. Even in the final moments before I succumbed to the first whiffs of anesthesia, I instinctively retained the part of me that was still just a young woman who, in addition to feeling frightened and alone, was also self-conscious about her exposed body: how it must look to the people in the bleachers who gazed down at her as they flipped open the top of a Coke can or stuffed another piece of gum between their teeth.

I was on display. My transplant was going to be a great big show.

"We've got the heart here!" The voice of a doctor shot out from behind a swinging door.

"She's all set. Let's go."

Curtain up. My cue.

Terrified, I took my place on the stage set for my heart transplant.

Mine was not the only awful pre-surgery moment to occur that night. There was another as well, that had unfolded just a few hours earlier in a different operating room, on a different body, not just miles but states away from New York's Columbia-Presbyterian Hospital. I was to have the second mind-blowing surgery of the evening; the first one having been performed on a thirteen-year-old girl who lay brain-dead in an Ohio hospital. She was to be the donor of a pair of healthy lungs, a liver, two kidneys, and a heart that would soon become mine.

I wasn't supposed to know anything about this young girl, my organ donor. Anonymity was the clearly stated—but more than occasionally circumvented—rule in 1988, years before more specific and highly policed privacy regulations came into effect. Absolutely no information was to be divulged about the donor, the donor family, the circumstances of the donation, or even the number of hours the donated organ had spent "on ice"—that is, in a cooler during transport from donor to recipient (many patients were aware of the evidence that shorter "ice" periods made for more successful transplants). The rules surrounding donor anonymity would often have their limits pushed to the very edges in the late 1980s, if only unintentionally, because of the heady enthusiasm that frequently infected doctors on transplant teams, who would be sent on emergency missions by helicopter, airplane, or ambulance to retrieve lifesaving organs. By the time doctors arrived back at their hospital of origin, carrying the type and size of cooler more often used for a six-pack of beer at picnics (but this one with the words ORGAN FOR TRANSPLANT written in black Magic Marker across the side panel), they could hardly contain their excitement. It was almost expected that he or she might run off at the mouth, break a rule or two, and give the recipient's family what they asked—or begged—for, firsthand donor information.

"She died in a car accident—a thirteen-year-old girl. Ohio."

The retrieval doctor blurted out this prohibited information to my parents on the night of my surgery. He was breathless as he spoke, as if he'd just run the last bit of the distance from Ohio to New York instead of flying on the medical plane. "Took it out myself. A great heart. It's very healthy. Young."

And so, sometime after waking from surgery I came to know—in spite of the rules—at least a few important details about the donated heart that had been placed in my chest after my own had been removed. But I always tried to keep in mind that, in the absence of documentation, nothing was for sure. I was, perhaps, less eager to believe a happy donation story than other patients, certainly less eager than one unnamed patient in particular, whose story stood out among the gossip that buzzed through the transplant clinic. This patient, a kidney recipient at another hospital, ended up a victim of donor misinformation, the consequences of which were nothing short of a transplant shame. On the night of his surgery, there had been another transplant (a heart) done at the same hospital. After receiving his new kidney, the patient asked for information about the donor and was told it was a man who had worked most of his life as a chef. Feeling tremendous gratitude, the patient changed his will to leave the bulk of his money to a culinary school in honor of the organ donor who saved his life, and years later, when the kidney patient died, much of the value of his estate was transferred to the culinary school, just as he'd directed. A gift had been returned in kind.

Or so he thought. As it happened, the donor of his kidney had not been a chef at all; the many years of cooking had in fact been done by the donor of the *heart*—the one that was placed in someone else on the same night. The transplant staff became aware of the misinformation after the fact, but the new and more stringent privacy regulations prevented them from setting the kidney patient straight. The poor guy didn't have a chance; even if he had made further inquiry, no one would have told him the truth.

Had my parents been told the truth?

"Which city in Ohio?" my father asked, attempting to pull another detail out of the ebullient doctor who'd fetched my donor heart. Maybe he'd oblige.

Dayton was the answer.

But who could say for sure? The small details of any heart transplant will always hold a bit of uncertainty, if not insoluble mystery. A slice of wonder inevitably goes with each of the steps and stages in the transfer of a vital organ from one body to another. And a hint of the unknowable will always linger.

Take, for instance, the intriguing reports from newly transplanted patients who claim they feel more than just an infusion of life with their new organs; they find themselves strangely and irresistibly attracted to certain foods or styles of music in their post-transplant lives. Hard put to explain this, they come to the conclusion that these particular tastes belonged to their donors and must have been transplanted into the bodies along with the new organs.

In the years after my surgery, I would come across magazine articles featuring transplant recipients whose lives were transformed by what they believed was the infusion of the sensibilities of their organ donors into their own bodies. One man claimed that his new kidney was filled with Frank Sinatra music; having never liked the crooner before his surgery, now he couldn't get enough of "Fly Me to the Moon." And a woman told how she came to adore anything pickled—cucumbers, beets, herring—after her liver transplant. Both patients reported their newfound tastes as an urge that called out from somewhere deep inside. Lacking any evidence that transplanted kidneys or livers carried anything more than tissue, blood, and vessels with them in their journey from body to body, doctors were quoted in one article as attributing the reported phenomena to the elation that transplant recipients feel after their surgery. It was no surprise, they said, that a transplant patient might develop new tastes or other sense inclinations after receiving a healthy new organ—given the natural propensity to get so darned filled up with all that post-transplant gladness, of course.

I never experienced even the smallest change in my food or music preferences. Sure, I awoke from surgery with a sense of peace that harkened back to my days as a normal healthy woman, and I experienced momentary euphoria before drifting back to sleep, but this was short-lived. If I thought the sensation of quiet in my chest was any indication of the life I would have after my transplant, I was sorely and swiftly disappointed.

14

Nurse Vera made me brush my teeth. Worse than that, she made me stand up at the sink and do it. Just two days after my transplant, I found myself at the mercy of a petite sinewy woman in white, with tight cornrows lining her scalp and a no-nonsense lower lip that protruded threateningly at the first sign of my reluctance to follow her orders. There were only two things on Nurse Vera's mind—getting me out of bed, and keeping me out as long as possible—and she went about making these happen with an insistence that, I thought at the time, bordered on a Nurse Ratched brand of sadism.

But I was wrong about Vera.

"You stand there now, girl, and brush those teeth!" she hammered.

I swayed in front of the edge of the sink and nearly toppled over before she caught hold of my arm.

"Come on. None of that weak stuff. Brush your teeth. You're a grown girl!"

"Oh, please. . . . Can't I just get back into bed? I feel awful . . . so weak. . . ."

"Brush 'em!"

I brushed. Whimpering with each lethargic pass of the toothbrush over my gum line, I stood in front of a bathroom mirror for the first time in almost two months and did as I was told. Because Vera said so.

"Good girl," she told me, more like an order than an accolade. "Now you're going to sit in the chair."

Sit in the chair? Cruel!

"Ten whole minutes, and not a second less, you hear?"

Impossible!

After the third minute I began to slump.

"Up, up, up! You gotta sit there now. A chair's not for lyin' down!"

I sat, disappointingly more down than up. Soon, giving in to unbearable weakness, my chin fell onto my chest, and I began to cry without tears; the whining had kicked in again.

Nurse Vera was unimpressed. She stood beside me like a sentry with her arms folded over her chest, eyes staring straight ahead at the blank wall—except for the occasional glance downward at her watch.

"Time's up," she said finally, without emotion. "You *can* sit yourself up in a chair, girl. You see that now?"

She placed her forearm beneath mine and guided me the few steps back to my hospital bed. I noticed that at some point between teeth cleaning and chair sitting, Vera had managed to smooth my sheets and blanket, turn them down neatly, and fluff both my pillows.

I slid beneath the sheets and lay back in the comfortable softness.

"Remember, none of that weak stuff now. You hear?"

I'd heard loud and clear. And so, apparently, had Vera heard me. She had only been my ICU nurse for a few days, but already she'd managed to gain insight into the post-transplant woman who'd come under her constant watchful eye: this heart-transplant girl was a fighter with a will and a spirit that were plenty powerful—in spite of all that silly whimpering. Vera understood that I was not a patient who would take too well to supportive coddling or to slow, easy, tiny steps forward. True, I was a young woman who had been weakened by a sick heart, but I had only been ill for a short time (extremely short for a transplant patient). The best thing for me, Vera knew, was to get back to normal as soon as possible and regain my independence before I'd forgotten it entirely. This meant giving me the legs I needed to get out of the ICU. In her wisdom and stubborn will, Vera knew instinctively to put my recovery on the fastest exit track she could in her capacity as a critical-care nurse. She pushed me up and out—for my own good—and refused every step of the way to treat me like the other heart-transplant patients.

I was far from typical in the post-transplant ICU. The majority of patients who came through her unit were men in their fifties or sixties who had undergone transplant after suffering years of progressively debilitating heart disease that had made a normal life impossible for them. These patients percieved a heart transplant as a welcome solution, a godsend, even if it meant accepting a severely truncated life span that would undoubtedly be filled with immunosuppression-induced infections and serious secondary illnesses, like cancer, kidney failure, and diabetes. At least their hearts were okay, if only for now and the next few years; this was what mattered most to a patient who, having lived with heart disease for a long time, was getting a second shot at life—a transplant! Now the lucky guy could go out and play nine holes of golf again, go fishing with his grandson, even get behind the wheel and drive to the drugstore.

This was the kind of grateful chatter I would hear at the transplant clinic in the weeks, months, and years after my surgery. Intermingled with complaints about post-transplant ailments, there were also dewy-eyed claims by these same patients that their new hearts had given them their lives back. This was my signal to remain silent and disappear behind a magazine. Sometimes I'd even walk out of the clinic into the hallway, just to get away from the terrible feeling that I was the lowest, most ungrateful transplant patient ever. Because I felt my heart transplant had taken my life away.

I never felt the sense of relief most heart-transplant patients experience when their surgery frees them from years of incapacitating illness. The evolution of my heart problem from a diagnosis of cardiomyopathy to transplant surgery spanned just eight months; I had lain in a hospital bed for only seven weeks of this time—at the very end. This was not long enough to make me staunchly, unalterably grateful for my transplant. To me, it was not great just to be alive; I wanted to be cured. I wanted to have my healthy, carefree life back as I knew it—just as it had been before that Black Monday when everything came crashing down on me in Dr. Bradley's office. And that day was not so far back in time that I had forgotten what it was to be a well person; I could still recall quite clearly how *normal* felt. The more typical transplant patients, whose long battles with heart disease had allowed the contours of healthy living to fade from memory, were—I was ashamed to think—better off.

And in my shame at my transplant ingratitude, sometimes I would turn my thoughts to the thirteen-year-old girl whose natural-born heart was now inside my chest, and I'd wonder if she would think me disgustingly ungrateful as well. Here I was—alive—my every breath made possible only through her tragic death, and I was the one complaining. Would she hate me for it? Would she regret that her precious heart had not been given to someone who would truly appreciate it?

Sometimes I'd ask her, in silence. And the spirit of my transplanted heart would be there to answer, a nurturing female aura hovering close to my chest, listening, watching, and experiencing transplant life right along with me. When I needed to, I would allow myself to believe that this faint presence was in fact the young girl who had given me her heart, and I imagined that she looked on with compassion, not at all disappointed in me for failing to show sufficient gratitude. She saw how I tried and tried to be a well person; she also saw me fail time and time again. Her presence was there in each and every heartbeat, warm, knowing, and encouraging. At moments, it would strike me as spooky and sad that a deceased thirteen-year-old girl would understand my heart-transplant body better than anyone else ever would.

She'd answer me in the circulating of my blood; in the quick pulsing beneath my once-severed ribs: *No, no, no,* the unspoken voice told me with each beat. She wouldn't want her heart to live on in any other chest but mine.

After just five days under Vera's care, I was sufficiently sturdy to move down to the hospital floor designated for newly transplanted patients. I didn't know about the freedoms and the joys that awaited me there; for the first time during my hospitalization, almost all the surprises would be pleasant ones.

The first came my way just minutes after I was rolled into my new room on a stretcher: a nurse came by to remove my IV. She withdrew the small needle from my forearm, very matter-of-fact, but to me the impact was tremendous because I hadn't been without intravenous medicine since landing in the emergency room in Philadelphia. No longer attached to an IV pole, I was now able to move about freely—and with my new healthy heart I could walk up and down the hall unassisted, whenever I liked. I could also start wearing my own clothes again, since the easy emergency access of a hospital gown was no longer necessary; I put on a T-shirt and sweatpants for the first time in almost two months. And there was another lovely surprise: when it came time to take my morning medicines—more than a dozen of them—I was allowed to set them up by myself, counting out pills from bottles while a nurse supervised from a distance. I was also in charge of my own food. No longer prisoner to whatever hospital meal arrived at my bedside, I was welcome to borrow takeout menus at the nurse's station and order in my first post-transplant pizza or chicken fried rice.

But the most wonderful of all the new liberties was the one situated directly across from my room: the shower. I could wash my hair and body under a stream of hot water for the first time since arriving at Columbia.

"I'm afraid my heart will stop or tear off or something," I told Beverly before heading for my first shower, fully aware of how ridiculous my words sounded as they hit the air but knowing that she wouldn't judge.

"I'm going into that shower room with you today, and I will sit there until you're done," she said.

"No, it's okay. I can do it myself. I don't *really* think my heart will tear off."

"Of course you don't. But it will be easier for you if I'm there. And you know I'm happy to do it."

I did know this—very well. It was something I appreciated every day on the transplant waiting list. Beverly had done so many things for me during my hospitalization, things that couldn't possibly have made her—or anyone in her place—particularly "happy." A few weeks ago, she had slept at my bedside in the ICU on a wooden chair; now she was just as happy to help again—with my first post-transplant shower—even if it meant having to deflect some undeserved angry-girl sass off the walls of a steamy bathroom. A spike in my fear and frustration was no match for her arsenal of optimism anyway.

I began to undress myself and then realized how badly my hands were shaking—partly from fear, partly from excitement, and also, perhaps, partly from my new medicines. My new doctor, transplant cardiologist Ron Davis, said the immunosuppressive drugs might cause tremor. He'd rattled off a long list of possible side effects; this particular one seemed less troublesome and so had escaped my mind—until now. Beverly noticed how hard it was for me to maneuver my T-shirt shirt up and over my head; without a word, she grabbed it from the top and helped me along.

Then I set out to slide off my sweatpants, one trembling leg at a time. Beverly allowed me to try to handle this challenge on my own. She pivoted away and turned on the shower water, testing it several times until the temperature was just right.

I baby-stepped in and looked down at my naked body. It had been a long time since I'd seen myself from this point of view, but I could tell at once that something was different. Something was wrong. My belly button was gone. Dr. Davis had warned me—in so many carefully chosen words—that the prednisone might do something like that. "Steroids may cause a bit of distension in the abdomen," he'd said, not knowing that I had recoiled from the mere mention of prednisone long before my transplant. Now I would have to take this drug for the rest of my life, and look what it had done to my body already, after only a few days!

My formerly washboard-flat stomach—which had always formed a slight curve inward between the span of my hip bones—had become a massive appendage. The indented space of my belly button had disappeared into the protruding spongy bloat without a trace.

"Beverly, come take a look at this!" I pulled the plastic shower curtain away from the wall and turned to the side so that she could get the most picturesque view of my prominent belly. "Looks like I'm in about my sixth month, wouldn't you say?"

"More like the third. But so what? Your body will get back to normal when the medicine levels come down."

I felt a sudden urge to curl up and weep. "Yeah? Meanwhile, I have to walk around with a frat-boy beer belly! Look at me!" I held my arms out to the sides and pivoted to face Beverly head on. "This is not my body!" I slid the curtain back across the rod in a huff, cordoning off my stepmother's calm positive viewpoint with a more apparent display of anger than I'd intended. *Oh, come on, Amy,* I thought to myself with immediate regret, once behind the shower curtain again; *give her a break.* I peeked out at Beverly through the slice of open space between the hanging plastic sheet and the wall. There she was, sitting low to the ground on an aluminum shower stool set off in the corner of the tiny hospital bathroom. She would spend the next ten minutes enduring thick steam and a heavy mildew smell along with me just so that I wouldn't feel nervous while standing beneath a stream of hot water that promised to cause all kinds of scary sensations in my post-surgery body. It was my first shower in a very long time, after all. It was also my first block of minutes in "active standing" since my surgery, and I was frightened by an array of possibilities that I thought might just happen to me under this steaming downpour that seemed so unfamiliar: I might fall over from dizziness, I might get disgusted to the point of nausea at the sight of my scar and pass out, or I might reach up to comb some conditioner through my hair and somehow cause my new heart to detach and drop down into my stomach!

Beverly remained calm. "You will get your body back the way you want it. You're young. You'll just have to eat right and start some kind of exercise routine, like walking or riding a bike." These were activities that, according to Dr. Davis, I would be able to do very soon. In a day or two, I was going to be taken from my hospital room down to the physical therapy suite, where I would walk at a good clip on the treadmill; after that, I'd bike. Exercise was close at hand, but the prospect of it was scary and I was annoyed by Beverly's upbeat take.

"We don't really know how I'll do at exercise yet, do we?" I snarled, ending my shower abruptly. I turned off the water for better acoustics and huffed a few times for effect.

Unfazed, Beverly held her arm out to me as I stepped over the rim of the tub and onto the tile floor. I needed that arm; there was not a part of my body that wasn't quivering with exhaustion and medicine by then. Arm in arm, we navigated a few small slow steps to the stool where Beverly had been sitting, sweating in the steam, for the last twenty minutes. I threw down a towel, gave in helplessly to the intense shaking of my quadriceps, and dropped my rear end onto the seat with an uncontrolled thump.

"Do you want me to get the nurse?" Beverly asked.

"No, I'm okay. Just weak. I'm glad you're here, Bev. Thanks." I had given up the fight against her happy talk—for now, at least.

Beverly wasn't done with her cheerleading, though, and I was a captive audience, slumped on a tripod stool. She looked down at my belly while draping a second towel across my shoulders and then picked up where she'd left off. "Really, Amy. You're exaggerating about your stomach. It's practically nothing—not nearly as big as you think. And it'll go away soon enough. I really wouldn't worry about it."

That was Beverly for you, always with an upbeat outlook and never a worrier. Not about a prednisone potbelly, not about raging heart viruses, and not about transplant survival statistics either. Beverly didn't see the point of thinking about things too much. "It'll only make you upset," she'd say. "Why get upset when there's nothing you can do about it anyway?"

I knew in that post-shower moment—and would reflect on it for a long time to come—that someone like Beverly would make a much better transplant patient than I ever could. To be able to see a beach-ball stomach as being just barely a little curve in the belly: that's the kind of antiworry viewpoint—or healthy denial, really—that makes for a happier heart-transplant life. To easily assume and truly believe that a bit of exercise and some moderate changes to one's diet will combat the powerful side effects of high doses of prednisone: that sure is a positive worry-free way to orient one's mind, even if the idea is, admittedly, couched in a pipe dream. And to find a way to make a decision—a firm commitment, if necessary—to eschew all worry, especially about what might go wrong in a heart-transplant body: that would be the key to achieving the optimum level of post-transplant peace of mind. It is the kind of commitment that demands sturdy courage, because right alongside the irksome problems like prednisone potbelly there will always be the high risk of death from a variety of transplant-related causes. Without the inner strength to do away with worrying, death sits like a monkey on the heart-transplant patient's back.

But not on Beverly's. Perhaps if she'd had a heart transplant, she would sail on through, easy-breezy—straight to her grave, if it must be—smiling every minute of the ride, a model patient with just the right attitude for inner peace.

I was a very different kind of patient.

Because I thought too much. And thinking too much leads to knowing too much. And knowing too much would make it impossible for me to live in carefree denial. So I would worry or, as I saw it, I would ponder, I would question, and I would take extra precautions, in all the places another patient might not. I refused to dive into my heart transplant life worry free and with my eyes closed. I couldn't help but think—and figure, and ruminate, and calculate—that by sticking to an intelligent, painstakingly honest self-assessment of my new heart and its problems, I might have the best chance of outsmarting the danger that loomed over me at all times: transplant-related death.

There was safety in planning and thinking and analyzing carefully.

For me, there had always been safety here, long before I lost my heart. From an early age, my unstable home life had forced me to think hard about how to survive it. By the time I was a teenager, I already had a plan in place: bide my time, keep my head down, and tread water until I was eighteen, when I could leave for college and never return to my mother's house. If I kept to my plan, in time I would have the life I wanted.

But the "think first" lesson had been taught to me earliest, perhaps in the telling and retelling of a favorite story—a parable my father would repeat with slight variations as I grew from child to girl to young woman. He would weave the tale into a conversation until he arrived at the last line, when he would pause—for effect and also to allow me to fill in the punch line—because the ending had a funny ring to it, almost like one of his jokes. And then he'd hit home the intended moral.

Lake Stupid was the final line. It had made me laugh when I was seven. As I got older, it made me think.

The story went like this: Long ago, on an Indian reservation that ran alongside a very wide and deep lake, there lived an Indian boy who fell in love with a beautiful girl far across the water. The boy had no canoe with which to paddle to his beloved, so one night he set out to reach her by swimming. This was a poor choice, as he knew he could hardly swim. But nothing would keep him from enjoying the happiness he anticipated on the other side of the lake; whatever it took, he'd be sure to claim for himself the love he believed to be his natural right. So the boy threw caution to the wind, plunged into deep water, and drowned. A ceremony was held in the village the next morning, and the wise chief made a pronouncement: "From now on this sacred lake will carry the name of the brave one who died in its waters. We will call it . . ." *pause* . . . "Lake Stupid."

Most times I would beat my father to the punch line.

Then he'd tell me, "Bravery and foolishness sometimes go hand in hand." Mere words to a seven-year-old. A veiled warning to a teenager. Vital wisdom to a twenty-five-year-old heart-transplant recipient.

My father's story came to mind my first night out of the ICU, when I found myself alone after dinner, back in an ordinary hospital room. Desperate to make sense of what had happened to me on that operating table, and aching for direction in a life that had been turned upside down and twisted into a daunting mess, I grabbed a pen and a yellow legal pad and set out to find safety in enumeration. I decided to make a careful deliberate list of my intentions, setting out exactly how I would live my life from that day on. It seemed to me I didn't need to know all the details of what I would face living with a heart transplant, I only needed to decide who I would be, and the only thing I had to base this decision on was who I had been before I got sick.

So I decided I would be normal.

I thought at the time that I was being entirely fair to myself. There had been a ten-year limit placed on my life expectancy with this new heart, plus warnings about how difficult the first year would be, living with high levels of immunosuppressive drugs and an ever-present risk of my body's rejecting my new heart, but no doctor had explained to me just how I was supposed to live out my ticking clock. Besides the daily mound of pills and the twice weekly heart biopsy appointments, I was left to fill in the blanks of my new post-transplant life on my own. It felt only natural to fill them with the strength of mind and will that had marked my personality before I landed on the heart-transplant waiting list. My ultimate desire was to shape my heart-transplant life along the lines of how I'd lived the twenty-five years leading up to my surgery: surviving a difficult childhood with a combination of smarts, courage, and patience; delving into academic life with joy while achieving the highest honors; and managing to keep a menacing heart illness as far away as I could from my law school studies and the love between me and Scott.

But if I willed myself to continue this way, would I be diving into my new life like the Indian boy into the lake?

Time spent living with a transplanted heart would soon show me that trying to maintain my pre-transplant way of life would only cause perpetual self-torment and frustration. It turned out that to make myself "normal" again would be a most extraordinary feat that I could never quite accomplish. So with all my resolve spilled out onto the lines of a yellow pad, I tumbled unknowingly into the long hard fall that would come to be my heart-transplant life. Like the headstrong Indian boy, I would drown in my own will.

15

A YOUNG WOMAN NAMED ELLEN WAS MY INSPIRATION FOR ONE OF the intentions I scratched out on my pad: *I will not be like other transplant patients.*

A nurse suggested that I take a walk down the hall and have a chat with this "super gal" who'd also had a heart transplant in her twenties, just like me. Only—well, Ellen had undergone two heart transplants. Maybe three. Or was it four? The nurse wasn't sure at the moment; she was busy counting out the fourteen pills that I would soon have to swallow. No matter. There were other things to tell me about Ellen, things she was more certain about: little enticements that would prod me to initiate a visit with the stranger down the hall. Ellen's age was right around mine, she said, and wasn't it a strike of luck that she just happened to be here today, on the same hospital floor, right at the time when I was recovering from surgery? Surely we'd have lots to talk about, with so much in common. I should go now—right now, the nurse said—and seek out my young friend-to-be, because there was no way she would be coming in my direction anytime soon. Ellen wasn't allowed to get out of bed.

This was because she'd just had her "annual exam," which consisted of a heart biopsy and a coronary angiogram. Since the angiogram involved cutting into an artery in her groin, Ellen had to spend the next six or seven hours lying on her back while the incision healed and clotted sufficiently well.

I replaced my pajama bottoms with a pair of sweatpants and headed out of my hospital room, ready to meet face-to-face with my very first transplant peer—someone supposed to be just like me.

And at first glance, it seemed that she was.

Even lying flat on her back in a hospital bed, Ellen had the distinctive appearance and outward indications of a normal, active woman in her twenties. Her hair was shiny and well cut, her nails recently polished—I could tell—and she wore a pair of stretchy exercise pants that looked just like the ones I'd left behind in my law-school dorm room. On the small table beside her bed were some of the same magazines that had piled up on mine—*Glamour, Self,* and *People*—plus a small container of Blistex. There was a ringing telephone that she answered with a lighthearted "Hey there! I'm great! How are you doing?"

Ellen could have been me. Or I, her.

She sensed it too, I thought. She was immediately welcoming, offering me a piece of Dentyne and some Milanos, along with the promise of an undiluted play-by-play account of her heart-transplant history. It was just the kind of openness that I myself might offer to a young heart-transplant woman who'd wound up at my bedside in awkward search of commonality. There was something about sharing the same absurdly rocky boat of heart transplantation that made sharing the details of one's medical history seem natural and right, if a bit strange.

We were on our way to a transplant friendship. A bond, I thought.

At first.

Then Ellen told me her story. She'd developed heart failure suddenly. It seemed to have come from out of nowhere; one day she was playing tennis and the next she couldn't lift her arm to serve without gasping. Her doctor thought that by resting her heart—with medications and the use of a wheelchair—Ellen might be able to turn back the progression of her cardiomyopathy, and he was right. Within six months, her heart function had improved enough so she could leave the wheelchair behind. Ellen returned to her daily life, much better but not yet cured. And she got pregnant.

I was shocked to hear this, Ellen could tell.

She waved a dismissive hand at me. "I know, I know. Why did I get pregnant, right? Well, we just thought, 'Let's go for it!' We figured it would be okay. But it wasn't, I guess."

Ellen's heart was unable to withstand the demands of pregnancy and deteriorated rapidly up until the day she gave birth to her daughter, when it simply gave out. An immediate transplant was necessary, and Ellen went straight from the delivery room to the transplant operating room to receive the first donor heart to become available that day. It was not a good tissue match. Her body rejected the new heart right away and Ellen went into a coma.

"Couldn't see my baby for days. Couldn't hold her, you know?" she told me.

I nodded, unable to speak.

Ellen went on to tell me about her second transplant, which followed her first by only a few days. She needed another heart again, her third, just a year or so later. Transplant artery disease had done its dirty work on heart number two, uncommonly quickly and furiously

Hadn't the nurse told me there had been a fourth transplant as well? No, it was only three. I'd lost my concentration to a sudden wave of nausea. How many heart transplants could one girl endure? How many donor hearts was a patient entitled to receive?

"So now I'm here for my annual exam on this one"—she turned her chin to the side and gestured toward the space above her left breast—"and I think everything is going to check out okay. This one's a keeper."

"It better be, 'cause they're sure not giving you another one."

I looked up and saw a wry smile on the face of her husband, Bob, who'd just spat out these words. Even in the dull flat lighting of the hospital room, Bob kept his dark Ray Ban sunglasses pressed far up on the bridge of his nose, making it impossible for me to see the expression in the eyes behind this remark. He leaned back against the wall with his arms crossed over his chest, clacked his Dentyne, and flipped some blond hair to the side with a quick toss of his well-cut jaw. This was the man—the husband—who was a full partner in willing his wife to get pregnant while she had cardiomyopathy. I wondered if Bob had taken off his fancy sunglasses and seen the light of day when he supported that decision.

Ignoring her husband's comment, Ellen went on. "So, as you can see, I know a whole lot about heart transplants here at Columbia. I can tell you plenty. First, you should know they're going to say that you can't get a handicapped license plate. But you can; I know how. It's kind of a transplant perk, and why not? You know, I once got the cable guy to come to my house on the same day I called for an appointment, because I told him I'd just had a heart transplant and I really, *really* needed my cable up and running. Isn't that right, honey?"

Bob lifted his chin up once and dropped it down: a cool Ray Ban–covered version of a yes.

"You might as well use your transplant any way you can," Ellen chirped.

What? A handicapped parking permit? Ellen had been the first to mention the prospect to me, but in the weeks ahead I would hear other patients talk about how they planned on filling out their applications for permits as well. I sensed an undertone of pride in their voices, as if a parking permit were a badge of honor. But I knew the moment Ellen had raised the issue that I would never use my heart transplant as an excuse to seek out handicapped parking privileges. I would feel proud of myself only for walking the distance from the farthest spot in the lot.

I held my tongue. It would be a loss to separate myself from the new "friend" I'd just made on the inpatient floor. Ellen was, sadly, all I had in the social world who was anywhere close to being me. Jumping on Ellen's transplant-wisdom bandwagon with a smile and a fib, I pulled myself back from the judgmental sidelines and told her, "Great. I'll have to remember that."

Ellen went on to tell me about other transplant maneuvers that she'd used to her advantage, like cutting down the number of required heart biopsies; not in a significant or dangerous way, but just shaving off one or two heart-snipping torture rides every now and then. She'd figured out between her second and third transplant that she could let a few of those nasty biopsy appointments slide and still be all right. It was also possible, she said, to "work your doctor" so that you could decrease your immunosuppressive medications before the prescribed date. I noticed the almost boastful glimmer in her eyes as she explained to me how she'd persuaded her doctor to allow her to stay home with an infection when he really would have preferred the safety of a hospital admission. What a coup.

These were the little victories that allowed Ellen to push aside the terrible nuisance that was her heart transplant. And Bob seemed to support risking Ellen's life in return for a little more of his own.

"Here's my number. Call me if you have any questions or anything." She tore off the corner of a piece of paper and handed it to me. "And maybe we can go out sometime. Have dinner."

"That would be fun," I said noncommittally. But as the years passed, Ellen and I only saw each other at transplant clinic. Occasionally, we'd talk on the phone; our conversations consisted mostly of transplant commiseration. Sometimes Ellen would pass along helpful tips, like how best to swallow cyclosporine (a liquid form of immunosuppressive medication that tasted like sulfur mixed with rancid olive oil) without gagging. There would be some dishy hospital gossip for me as well, which would lead to a few good laughs, and then the conversation would end—as always—with one of us saying, "We really should get together with the guys for dinner one night."

After more than a year of false starts, we found ourselves—two couples—walking down Christopher Street in the direction of a café in Greenwich Village, with Ellen and me in front and Bob and Scott just steps behind us. I could hear Bob's voice pounding at the back of my head, harsh and filled with sarcastic anger. It occurred to me that he might be drunk already.

"Hey, so how you doin'?" he asked Scott. "Wow, I mean, Ellen got sick after I married her, so I sort of had to, you know, take her with the transplant and all that. But you"—he was yelling now—"you weren't even married, for Christ sake! Why'd you do it, man?"

I continued walking, not looking back to see Scott's reaction. He told me in bed later that night that he thought Bob was "an unbelievable asshole." Then he took me in his arms and mumbled something about how he never would have let my heart transplant stop him from marrying me. Not in a million years. "He doesn't love her the way I love you."

Scott must have been right about that. Bob divorced Ellen a year later.

Soon afterward, Ellen died. She'd battled her doctor once again not to be hospitalized—this time for a bad cough that seemed to be headed for some kind of upper respiratory infection. By the time she coughed her way through the doors of Columbia's emergency room, the infection was already too far gone. I had seen Ellen at transplant clinic just two days before. She'd told me there—through wheezes and hacking—that life in her body was getting her down: all those transplants and the high levels of medicine she had to take in order to protect her heart. And to make it worse, she said, her ex-husband was a rat. But still, there was one pure joy: her six-year-old daughter. She said her favorite part of every day was when she lay down with her at bedtime and sang quietly, "You've Got a Friend," each refrain of the chorus reminding her that here, with her arms wrapped around this little girl, she had the only friend she would ever need.

I saw Ellen's daughter at the funeral, dressed in a velvet-trimmed navy jumper with patent leather shoes to match. She played a running game on the lawn outside the temple until it was time to come in and then stood beside her father, who again left his dark sunglasses on, even inside the dimly lit sanctuary. I did not care to see the eyes behind them this time.

The rabbi said that Ellen had lived a blessed and rich life in spite of her "health challenges," and that her strength and spirit had touched us all. "Ellen's is a soul that will not soon be forgotten," he bellowed, lifting his arms to the sky for effect, "not in our minds and not in our hearts."

I shuddered and let my face drop into my hands. Not soon be forgotten? Ellen had undergone three transplants at Columbia and spent many years as an ever-present patient there, but nobody from the transplant team showed up at her funeral. I imagined there might be rules against that kind of display of involvement with a patient; yet it seemed odd that there was not one face from Columbia—not one—willing to show itself for Ellen. How quickly every one of her long-term doctors, nurses, physical therapists, social workers, nutritionists, and transplant blood technicians had moved on.

The rabbi was reframing Ellen's life for the consolation of others: Ellen was happy and content; a mother, a contributing member of the community, a member of this temple; Ellen was fortunate; Ellen was hopeful, bright, and optimistic about her life; Ellen would not have wanted us to be sad today.

I buried my nose deep into a wad of tissues. It was all I could do not to cry out, *You've got to be kidding! Ellen was sick nearly every day of her transplant life! She hated it! And her husband bailed on her!*

Poor Ellen, I thought: lying there dead and unable to save the story of her post-transplant life from the rabbi's contortions. How many people sitting in the audience that day knew the truth about what she'd suffered, transplant after transplant after transplant? Ellen had endured endless illnesses, many of them exacerbated by her successive heart transplants and high levels of immunosuppression. Sometimes she'd call me on the phone and say how hard it was for her, and I could hear in her sighs the creeping destruction of the carefree Ellen I'd once known. One of these calls came in the wake of a strep infection that had invaded a spot on Ellen's leg where a tiny mole had been removed; her body had become flooded with rampant infection, nearly killing her, all because the damn transplant medicines had shut her immune system down so dangerously.

Ellen had her chest cut open by a chain saw three times before she was in her early thirties. She'd had an insensitive selfish bore for a husband who nevertheless devastated her with his departure. It seemed to me that Ellen would want us all to feel more than just a little bit sad for her—a young woman who died after a long, hard, freakish fight and who'd left behind a child who would now be raised by a man she must have come to loathe.

And, again, where the hell was everyone from Columbia? Didn't she mean anything to them?

Wouldn't I mean anything to them?

At that moment, Ellen's funeral could easily have turned into a model for my own. What happened to her could very well happen to me: immunosuppression, infection, death. We were both young women with heart transplants who tried to live normal lives the best we knew how. But even as I drove my car away from the funeral site, I was sure that this was the point at which our similarities came to an end. I was already separating from Ellen, reassuring myself that, in truth, we had lived our transplant lives very differently. I needed to believe that our transplant deaths would be different as well.

So I thought back on the night of the ill-fated couples dinner we'd shared at that Greenwich Village café. Ellen had downed two gin and tonics (alongside her husband's vodka martinis) before the appetizers arrived. Oh, she was a brave one, that Ellen. Right before my knowing, judging eyes, she fearlessly broke the rules: heart-transplant patients are not allowed to drink any alcohol—except for a single drink on a special occasion, like a wedding or an anniversary. When Ellen gave the waiter her drink order—after I'd asked for club soda with lime (I did not have a drop of alcohol or wine in the seventeen years after my transplant)—she affirmed her determination not to act like a heart-transplant patient and live in deference to her health issues. She adamantly refused to coddle her body, declaring she would treat it (or abuse it) just like any "normal" person might.

"You can drink, you know," she said to me that night.

"Oh, I know. I just don't."

"But you can," she repeated, gazing down into the nearly empty cocktail glass in front of her.

"Sure," I said, feather light, thinking I could also skip my next heart biopsy but would not.

Lake Stupid, I thought.

The interweaving of bravery and foolishness: yes, my father had spoken wisely if not prophetically. Ellen was not afraid of her body, and this had made her brave but also foolish, given the realities of her heart-transplant life. Perhaps a healthy dose of fear might have won her a few more years with her daughter, perhaps not. One thing was for sure, though: Ellen's brave denial allowed her to live a more normal life than I ever would. For all the hard work and brain-busting thought I put into surviving my transplanted heart, Ellen looked for ways to slack off and enjoy. For every disagreeable rule in Columbia's transplant handbook that I followed to its farthest point, there was one she broke with defiant glee. Ellen would never write down her firm intentions on a yellow legal pad the way I had done. She didn't need to commit herself to a set of high expectations in a desperate effort to hold on to the person she was before her transplant; she simply remained that person. It was as if she never for a moment feared that her heart transplant would make her into someone else. Or that it would kill her—so suddenly—with a cough gone awry.

16

I WILL NOT LIVE SCARED.

It was one thing to jot down an intention like this one in tiny blue letters while sitting comfortably in the medically supervised safety of my hospital room. It was quite another to live it on the streets of New York City, where I would have to move through time and space with a heart that was new to my body and didn't feel at all like mine.

With my wedding date set for the following June, I had less than a year's time to shake myself loose from post-transplant fears. I had only eleven months, to be exact: summer to fall, winter to spring, and then Scott and I would marry at the Pierre. The following September, I would return to law school, finish my third year of studies, and sit for the bar exam. But today, a little more than a week after my discharge from the hospital, I would have to take one of those terrifying self-imposed walks—alone—out the door of my apartment building, past the mailbox on the corner, and then around half a block to the bakery. I would buy a quarter pound of assorted cookies there and return home. In previous days I had covered three other stores closer in distance (Korean market, wine store, newsstand). If I could do the bakery, I would surpass yesterday's yardage and meet my goal for the new day. And then I'd immediately have to set a more daunting objective for tomorrow: walk across Sixth Avenue and into the grocery store.

It would mean having to wear one of the masks a nurse had given me before I left the hospital. She had warned me about the dangers of being a newly transplanted, immunosuppressed patient caught in a crowd of germy New Yorkers. At the movies or in any closed-in space with a potentially germ-carrying population, I was supposed to tie a surgical-type mask across my nose and mouth so I might avoid "serious complications."

"Like what?" I'd asked her.

"Like a cold—even that would be dangerous for you right now. Something as simple as a stomach virus could be very bad. When you're out and about, you'll definitely want to put on that mask."

But I didn't want to at all. The mask only reminded me that there was yet another hovering health risk that called out for my fear; the most ordinary of activities (food shopping) might land me in the hospital. And wearing a surgical mask in public, among chatty New Yorkers who thought nothing of commenting on such anomalies with a rude sense of entitlement, would make me feel like an even bigger freak than my puffy prednisone face already did.

The next day, I put on the mask and passed through the sliding doors of the neighborhood A&P, thankful they'd opened in front of me automatically without my having to touch them with my hands.

I'm not a germ phobe! I wanted to shout. *I have to wear this mask because I had a heart transplant ten days ago. Yes, I'm a young woman with a heart transplant! I'm only afraid of your germs because I have to be. You don't know it, but I can die from a simple cold.*

Or maybe I could put a sign on my back: HEART TRANSPLANT PATIENT. DOES NOT SUFFER FROM OBSESSIVE-COMPULSIVE DISORDER. MUST WEAR PROTECTIVE MASK TO SAVE OWN LIFE.

I grabbed a shopping cart (*Remember not to touch contaminated hands to eyes before washing thoroughly*) and set out on my first post-transplant supermarket visit. Someone's sneeze over by the navel oranges sent me scurrying straight down the fruit aisle to the table at the end, skipping over the apples and pears I'd wanted to grab in between. The sound of a cough coming from aisle two told me to avoid that germ-ridden length of space altogether and caused me to forgo the two boxes of lasagna noodles and jar of sauce I'd needed to pick up for dinner. Scott would have to go back for them later.

Safety first.

I couldn't wait to get home so I could wash my hands.

And take my pulse.

Transplanted hearts practically call out for self-checks of pulse rhythm and rate. It's one of the secrets of heart transplantation that no one spoke of before I got out of the hospital (not even Ellen), but which everyone would confirm—if only reluctantly and in hushed tones—weeks later: transplanted hearts do not feel natural most of the time. They don't function normally either. The way they perform their vital pumping job is—as my doctors would later admit—simply "transplant normal."

Transplanted hearts like mine, I soon found out, cannot possibly beat normally because they have been cut off forever from the central nervous system. When I first heard this, I thought, Well, of course. When they took out my heart, all the nerves were severed. And when they took out the heart of my donor, her nerves must have been cut as well. It wasn't possible for Dr. Solomon to have reattached the bloody tangle of dangling nerve fibers.

Years later, one of the doctors explained to me that nerves are indeed cut and lost in a transplant recipient. All that is retained and reattached from the old heart is a piece of the atrium, the blood collection chamber. A transplant surgeon will always leave intact a small section of atrium from the recipient's heart so that he can use it as an anchor for the new atrium.

Not very normal at all.

What remains in the chest cavity of a heart-transplant patient, then, is a denervated heart with a nearly double-sized atrium that is missing its vital connection to the nervous system.

Without a nerve connection to transmit information on whether to speed up, slow down, or maintain status quo, a transplanted heart will wait for the flow of adrenaline to tell it what to do. So when a stimulus hits, like excitement, fear, or the sudden demands of exercise, the typical transplanted heart will flounder until a rush of adrenaline—often in overabundance—arrives. This constant dependence on adrenaline causes most transplant patients to have a very fast "resting pulse" (usually in the neighborhood of one hundred beats per minute), which can easily be set off into a racing gallop by any additional dump of adrenaline into the bloodstream.

I tried to explain the strange mechanism of my heartbeat—in the simplest terms I could—to an interested friend a few years after my transplant.

"It works this way: if you come up behind me and yell *boo! I'll* know you did it, but my heart won't—at least not at first. My heartbeat will remain at the same speed, even though you've just given me a scare. But a few minutes later, the adrenaline kicks in and my heart realizes it should be reacting to something, so it will start beating like wild—like there's nothing controlling it at all. Because there *isn't* anything controlling it, of course."

Of course?

How could my heart-healthy fully nerve-connected friend understand that?

She tried her best. "So you just have to wait a little while until your heart speeds up, that's all."

No. That's not all.

I have to talk to myself.

I have to bring my mind back from fear. I have to continue on with whatever I'm doing, even though my heart is off in some scary, crazy place. Because while the adrenaline begins to flood my veins, and my heart is still mindlessly, denervatedly pumping out its one hundred ignorant beats per minute, I feel like I'm going to die on the spot. My nerve-deprived heart gives me the terrifying sense of impending ventricular fibrillation. I feel it all the time, every day, every night; the baffled pump beneath my breastbone—my precious gift of life—reminds me over and over that, when it is asked to rise to an occasion, it has no idea what in hell to do. My body tries to tell it but can't. The signals fire and are never received. Then the adrenaline dumps, and there is upheaval. Suddenly I'm breathless. Or arrhythmic. I'm caught in a body that thinks it is climbing stairs, or thinks it is lifting a heavy basket filled with laundry, or thinks it is encountering a loud shout of *boo!* But, in reality, these events have already come and gone. My heart should have returned to a resting state, but instead it's riding high and wild on a tidal wave of adrenaline.

It was only natural that a denervated heart like mine would always command a fearful reaction.

But I'd committed myself to eliminating fear from my post-transplant life, and I set out to do it quick and clean on the crowded fast-paced sidewalks that lined lower Sixth Avenue. No excuses. Each day I hit the pavement of my testing ground and moved farther southward than I had the day before—legs wobbling from muscle atrophy and teeth chattering (even in the hot August sun) from the very fear I'd set out to conquer. Half a block, two blocks, ten blocks, fifteen: my denervated heart fought me every step of the way. *Stop, Amy,* it bellowed through my insides, taking my breath away, *something's wrong. You're asking too much of me. I might just have to quit beating if you continue on this way.*

But I wouldn't stop. There was a loving, supportive fiancé standing firm behind me, if only in spirit. Scott was my partner in fighting fear from the first day I returned home from the hospital. He wasn't going to let me stop either.

Six weeks later, my muscles had recovered enough for me to press on even farther. This time Scott led the way. "You can do it, up the hill! No resting! Just pick a spot and shoot for it. Don't stop till you've passed it by!" he huffed. We were race-walking. Scott was pushing me way beyond my comfort level; we weren't on our usual safe route—a city street that undoubtedly would have had a few CPR-trained policemen along its stretch or a neighborhood emergency room at the halfway point. No, today we were walking especially briskly in the suburbs near his mother's house, trekking along the steep hills and elongated inclines that had always seemed inconsequentially flat to me—until I tried to walk them with a transplanted heart.

"I don't feel right," I said, a few steps into our ascent. I'd spoken these same words to Scott from across the table in that Japanese restaurant in Philadelphia only a few months earlier; they'd landed me in the emergency room and under the defibrillator paddles. "My chest is tight. I need more air—slower air. I want to stop. I'm scared, Scotty!"

Scared.

One step backward in my fight against fear.

Scott refused to let me retreat. Without slowing the pace, he puffed out enough encouragement to keep me right there beside him, scaling the great hill of fear. "You have to remember—this is what hard exercise feels like. Even people without transplants get winded walking up a hill this fast. You just keep going. I'm here. Nothing is going to happen to you. Don't be afraid."

Together we made it to the crest of the hill and then down the other side. After my heart's initial delay in responding to the demands of the climb, adrenaline began its deluge. Soon my heartbeat was a spray of firecrackers inside my rib cage. Even when my pulse began showing the first signs of settling down, there would be only one word to describe how my heart felt thumping in the space beneath my chest wall: *wrong*. Little did I know that this feeling would become my new mind-bending *right* and I would spend the rest of my life trying to talk myself down from the fear it raised in me.

But today at least, it seemed, I'd achieved a victory.

I reached forward and grabbed hold of the back of Scott's gym shorts, pulling him into a moment of celebration between gasps of air. "Thanks for . . . pushing . . . me! . . . I can't . . . believe . . . I . . . did it!"

Breath. Breath. Breath.

Thump-thump-thump-thump-thump-thump-thump.

Scott swung around and placed his hands on my shoulders—a little bit out of breath himself, I noticed. "Of course you did it. You have a healthy heart now. There is nothing to be afraid of anymore."

At that moment, I believed him.

"Let's do it again!" I sang out, arms flailing, flying high on conquered fear.

So we did. Another hill and then another. Which led to longer hills a few weeks later, and faster ones in the months to come. Scott was my confidence, my rock—the voice of assuredness that could speak almost as loud as my unruly heart. I would carry his words with me into the future, as uphill climbs turned to bike rides and then to short jogs and finally to four-mile runs. Through all my post-transplant years, whenever I'd get ready to head out for some exercise, leaning over to pull on the laces of my sneakers, I would reach back for the memory I knew would carry me forward: Scott's steady, sure voice telling me, *You have a healthy heart now; there's nothing to be afraid of.* And again I would believe him: year after year, mile after mile, heartbeat after heartbeat. Scott's fearlessness would be the inspiration for my own.

Until the day came when I learned the truth about Scott's courageous confidence.

It was early on a spring morning nearly seventeen years after my transplant, and I'd just come in from my usual jog. Scott asked me how it had gone, and I told him (with a hint of do-you-really-have-to-ask?), "Much too hard. As always."

A swipe he didn't deserve.

"But you did it," he said, shrugging his shoulders.

Yeah, I did it, all right.

I stood with an open water bottle in my hand, still too breathless to take a sip. Scott smiled knowingly from over on the couch. He opened his arms out to the sides and gestured for me—panting, sweat-drenched mess that I was—to come take a seat on his lap.

"What?" I said, pretending not to know the meaning of the happy little crinkles that framed his eyes. "No, really. What?"

By now I had crossed the room and had come to a stop in the small space between couch and coffee table. Scott gave my arm a playful yank, and I collapsed onto his lap, laughing.

"You know, I was thinking about something this morning while you were out for your run," he said, turning suddenly serious. "I was remembering the first time you tried to exercise after the transplant. The first time we race-walked up that hill—together. Remember?"

I told him that I did and that I had been so scared.

"*You* were scared! How do you think *I* felt!"

I nearly jumped from Scott's lap. The uncharacteristic sharpness in his voice startled me. I couldn't quite make sense of his words: had Scott just asked me a question or was it more of a statement? I admitted to myself—with silent embarrassment—that if it had been a question, I didn't know the answer. I'd never given much thought to how Scott might have felt back on the day when he'd prodded me—his newly heart-transplanted fiancée—to climb a hill like a normal person.

Now for the first time I would understand the mind of the man who'd been my ever-confident coach; I would finally come to know the feelings hidden beneath the words of encouragement that had made possible my very first uphill trek. And today, with a post-jogging heap of heart-transplant success perched affectionately on his lap, Scott would feel free to tell all.

"What did I know?" he said, again with words that left me wondering whether Scott was asking or telling. "I had no idea whether you could make it up that hill or not. Dr. Davis never said I could push you so hard. It just felt to me—I don't know—like the right thing to do. And I was scared too, the whole time. You can't imagine what that was like for me."

He was right. I couldn't possibly imagine what it was like—because until this moment the whole concept of a fearful Scott had never occurred to me. It had always seemed that there was only enough room for one frightened soul in our relationship, and since I was the one who'd had my chest cut open, I thought it only natural that I should have first dibs on feeling terrified. I hadn't realized that even after all of my worries had been voiced, attended to, and coached away, Scott's still remained; they'd been there from the start.

And I hadn't noticed. Selfish, selfish me!

It seemed I'd let slip another one of the intentions I'd formulated just after my transplant: *I will never take Scott for granted.* When I wrote these words on my yellow pad, I did not expect that I would find myself seventeen years later stunned by the realization that I had overlooked and underappreciated one of the most extraordinary ways Scott had loved me throughout those years.

Scott had spared me all of his fears.

Only now did I recognize how hard this must have been for him. Scott had never been as free from worry as I had so blindly assumed. He was just in control of how he expressed it. I had always thought that love was all about communication and openness. But Scott had been showing me all along that the greatest love can sometimes exist in silence: in the pauses where one person chooses to carry a heavy burden alone, quietly and without resentment.

Scott had spared me—lovingly—so many times. I'd hardly spared him at all.

And now he was staring up at me, wide-eyed, from the couch, waiting for an answer I felt too ashamed to give.

"I didn't know you were scared," I said.

This wasn't nearly enough, for either one of us. Ignorance could not shield me from the newfound awareness that I'd taken Scott for granted. Another one of my post-transplant intentions had been completely washed out.

17

At seven o'clock in the evening on June 24, 1989, I stood in the center of an empty room waiting for Bella, my personal wedding dresser, to lower the Cinderella-style gown over my head. Bella steadied herself on the top rung of a stepstool, grabbed hold of the cloud of silk and tulle in gentle bunches, and dropped the huge hoopskirt from above in one fast motion, encompassing the whole of me in a world of white fabric that made a scratchy sound as it passed by my ears. Then she tugged softly from the bottom, nudging the gown past my shoulders and torso until it came to rest on my hips, where it took on a life of its own, flaring out from my small body with nearly three feet of hand-sewn finery. My wedding gown. I knew I would wear it only once, so I promised myself to try and remember every detail with precision: the way the intricate beaded material pulled tight across my waist, the heaviness of the long train spilling out behind me, and the swishing sound of the layered fabrics echoing in delayed response to my every move.

There was escape in this dress. There was so much more of it than there was of me. I could hide most of myself away from the nearly four hundred guests who would soon glance back over their shoulders in anticipation of my arrival. The sweeping movement of my gown down the aisle, alongside the tuxedo that held my father within its tailored formality, was not going to be just the forward motion of a young bride keeping step with the syncopated chimes of Pachelbel's Canon. The rows and rows of guests were going to witness much more than an exchange of vows. Tonight they would see a post-heart-transplant debut, something they had never seen before.

A few more minutes of final touches in the bridal dressing area—shoes, bracelet, earrings, veil—and I was whisked away to an anteroom. The whole day had been carefully orchestrated so that Scott would not set eyes upon me—or my gown—until Pachelbel's Canon morphed into the wedding march midway through my grand entrance into the ballroom. Now was the prescribed time for me to be alone, separated from the rest of the wedding party, who gathered in the hallway just outside my room. I positioned myself close to the wall and closed my eyes so I could concentrate on the sound of violins rising up each time the ballroom doors opened for the next member of the procession. I heard the doors close once again and the music disappear, replaced by the hum of anticipatory tension and the sound of muffled laughter. My father must have offered up a couple of jokes out there.

I turned away from the wall and opened my eyes, looking around me for the first time. This anteroom was actually another ballroom, much smaller than the one that hosted my wedding but just as ornate. On the ceiling, heavy gold-leaf trim surrounded an expanse of hand-painted mural: cherubs and angels set against a powder-blue sky. My eyes moved from the ceiling down to the walls. At the far end of the room I noticed the dim outlines of a person set back just beyond two marble columns. The light surrounding the mystery figure was barely one candle strong; I would have to squint my eyes and cock my head to the side for a moment before determining what—or who—was there with me in the anteroom. Then the image became clear: it was a bride.

No, it couldn't be! Was I going to have to share this room with someone else?

I stood frozen in disbelief before realizing, with a start, that there was in fact only one person here. The figure I'd glimpsed at the other end of the room was my own image reflected back at me in a floor-to-ceiling wall of antique mirror. With my entire form hidden beneath an enormous wedding gown and my face veiled, I saw only a vision: the quintessential bride. Not even a trace of sick girl.

The shadowy reflection was fairytale perfect—as long as I didn't move any closer to it. Any movement forward might change what I saw. With just ten steps toward the mirror I might be able to see the outline of my face beneath the veil—abnormally rounded and grossly distorted by the high doses of prednisone that were still part of my daily diet of medications. A couple of steps more and I would see a long crooked scar peeking through the delicate lace bodice that covered the center of my chest. Any closer, and the gold bracelet on my wrist would reveal itself to be the piece of jewelry it really was: a Medic Alert emergency information tag with the inscription *Heart transplant, on prednisone, cyclosporine, other medications*. I knew to stay put and admire this phantom bride from afar. It was the only way I could fix the image in my mind and carry it with me down the aisle. *Look, everyone,* it would say, *I'm not a sick girl anymore. I'm normal. Here comes the perfectly normal bride!*

The door to the room cracked open and my father popped his head inside. "Looks like we're up. You ready?"

"Sure, Dad."

"Then away we go!" he said, holding out an arm. We stood together in silence, a few feet back from the ballroom entrance. Two ushers waited for their cue to pull back the heavy doors, allowing for a pause before father and daughter stepped forward into the room.

"All right now, walk slowly and to the music," I heard someone say. Two panels of carved oak parted in front of me, revealing a Milky Way sky in the wonderland ballroom beyond. The entire ceiling had been covered in greenery, with tiny lights like stars woven into hundreds of hanging vines.

My body drifted along, skimming the length of the carpeted aisle as if on a light breeze. I walked without feet. I saw without eyes. I thought without connection to the familiar faces around me. My oversized gown and prominent veil would make my walk down the aisle feel, unexpectedly, like a solitary private moment. My mind turned inward and I followed it there, drifting away from my own wedding march. With each glide forward came another silent revelation: *One year ago on this same date, at this same time in the evening, I was on an operating table attached to a heart-lung machine.* The wedding date my father had set while I was on the transplant waiting list had been just a dream back then, and now it was coming true. Statistically, I wasn't supposed to have survived long enough to get a donor heart, but I did. I wasn't expected to complete my first post-transplant year without a single episode of rejection, but every one of my heart biopsies had come up uncommonly perfect. I hadn't been slotted by my doctors for running miles with a tricky transplanted heart, but I was now running almost daily. This moment—my wedding-aisle moment—became at once surreal; suddenly there were too many oddities caught beneath the draping of my veil, too many questions that had less to do with the padding along of my satin shoes on the wedding carpet than with the self-examination of my existence. *Why*, I asked myself, hiding away behind layers of whiteness, *am I alive?*

And how much of my being alive do I owe to luck? To Scott's love? To the skill of my doctors?

Wrapped in an elaborate cocoon of lace and flounce that separated me from the ogling guests beyond, I stumbled on an answer.

"*I* did it! *I* did it!" The silence beneath my veil was broken by words I hadn't meant to speak out loud. And here they came again: "*I* did it!" The sense of accomplishment swept me up; more than anyone or anything else, I was the force that carried my body through the dicey first post-transplant year and on to this wedding day. "*I* did it!" I must have repeated this to myself aloud a dozen times, but no one could hear me over the violins that sang out in unison from all four corners of the room. My words traveled only as far as my veil. No one could see my lips move or the tears as they flowed down to my chin, pooled there for a moment, and then dropped onto my chest. I did it! Life had pushed me all the way to the edge—maybe even beyond—but I had pushed back hard enough to stay alive. And now here I was, a woman in my mid-twenties, and I had discovered something few people glimpse in a whole lifetime: I had learned what I was made of.

I did it.

Holding my chin higher now, I continued my wedding promenade in front of hundreds of guests. I could see them grinning as I passed by, line after line of exaggerated smiles on the faces of people who didn't quite know what to make of me—this anomaly bride. It was at this moment that the oversized veil I'd picked out months earlier became my most treasured and useful wedding accessory. I may have felt a bride's love for the sweeping lines of my dress, the double-strand pearl bracelet, and the light blue ribbon that accented the garter around my thigh, but I was thankful only for my veil—the secreting, saving grace that delivered me down the long aisle. Because of this wonderful veil, I could hide my reality from a roomful of people.

I shifted my eyes to the left and spotted Susan, an old friend of Scott's who'd once asked me, "Do you have a monkey's heart?" Like everyone else in her row, Susan leaned all the way forward and craned her neck sideways so she could see the whole of my dress, from shoulder puffs down to the lacy hem. She turned away to face her husband for a moment, whispered something, and then swung around to gape at me again, this time laughing hard.

What's so funny, monkey-heart woman? I thought, safe beneath my veil. I should be laughing at *you,* you big dummy.

It had been just a few weeks after my transplant when she'd asked me where my heart had come from. I'd never met Susan before that; her husband had gone to grade school with Scott and we'd just now gotten together as couples for the first time, sort of a childhood reunion spread over lunch and an afternoon by the pool. In a manipulation intended to better acquaint me with the hostess, I was immediately named guacamole sous chef, and I stood beside Susan at the countertop, slicing limes and reading aloud from a recipe card. We were working nicely together; then came the question about my heart.

"No, no. Mine's not from a monkey," I said sweetly, trying not to make her feel bad for asking such a silly question. "Mine is from a girl who died in a car accident."

"Oh, so yours is from a person."

I told her yes, mine was, leaving open the possibility that someone else's transplant might very well have come from a chimp—or a goat, for that matter. To spare her embarrassment, I allowed Susan to believe it wasn't so much that she had been wrong, she was just—well, wrong about my particular heart, right?

And now here she was laughing at me, it seemed, as I walked down the aisle. If I had been more honest with Susan on the day we'd stood together amid the limes and tomato cuttings, if I had shot back at her the bold truth that monkey hearts were not being used in human beings and had never been used that way (so wherever did you get such an imbecilic idea?), she might not have found it so easy to let out an open cackle in the middle of my wedding march.

What did she know about my transplant anyway? What did anyone know?

I retreated beneath my veil again, continuing forward in measured steps. My eyes shifted from left to right, from face to face, all the while hidden. To my left, I could see a tuxedo-clad Dr. Ganz sitting beside his lovely wife. Down the row was an attorney from the law firm where Scott and I first met. Then there was a cousin I hadn't seen since I was thirteen. The next three rows were filled with friends: from grade school, college, law school, and work.

Sweeping my gaze over an even wider expanse of grinning guests, I was glad I'd decided not to invite anyone from the post-transplant team; it was the very absence of heart-transplant people in-the-know that allowed me to continue my picture-perfect ruse. I could straighten my spine beyond its natural line, pull taut the muscles of my upper back, and show off my best healthy-girl body language—small step by small step toward the altar.

It wasn't until I approached the final stretch of aisle that I focused on Scott, waiting for me at the end. There he was again, my beautiful boyfriend, my love, my angel man, this time in a formal tuxedo with tails. He stood, hands clasped in front of him, with a magnetic smile that penetrated the haze of my veil. His shining eyes locked on mine, pulling my thoughts into the spectacular reality of the present moment. This was not my post-transplant debut after all, it was my wedding. *Our* wedding. The grand show was over for now. Even if the curtain was still up, I wouldn't have to perform anymore. In this moment, I needed only to be Scott's bride.

I could tell by his captivated expression that I was just that: the woman he longed to love, honor, and cherish for the rest of his life. To be gazed upon by Scott at this moment was to be adored. No one else had ever looked at me the way he did as I approached the altar, and no one else ever would. Scott's eyes radiated a glow that was almost childlike: wide open, exaggerated, almond eyes that shone with a blend of curiosity and awe—the kind that comes with seeing your first shooting star or the perfect arch of a flying trapeze.

For Scott, there was no veil, no magnificent gown, no train of tulle flowing in my wake. There was only me, the real me. That's what Scott saw as I walked down the aisle: the unadorned truth. And still he was entranced, deep in love. Soon I would be standing beside this tuxedoed groom of mine; holding on to hands that could calm the tempest of a heart-transplant life.

Another few steps forward and a flicker of memory came to me: the words Scott had said in the hospital, just after a doctor had told us that one of my post-transplant medicines would be likely to cause tremors in my hands. I was immediately concerned and had reached out for Scott's reassurance. "What will I do when my hands start to shake so terribly—like this?" The tremors hadn't beset me too badly yet, but I was afraid they would soon enough. So I demonstrated for Scott what the shaking might look like in the future, setting my hands aquiver in front of his face.

"Then I'll just hold them . . . like this," he'd said, bringing my hands together in prayer position and enclosing them between his own, "and I promise I'll never let go."

Over the past year that had brought us to this wedding moment, that's just what Scott had done: he held on tight. Sometimes with his steady hands. Sometimes with the embrace of his arms. Sometimes with the sound of his voice through the telephone. Neither one of us could have anticipated all the ways I would need him to be there for me. How could we ever have imagined that Scott's promise to "never let go" would broaden in scope and require him to remain on the phone with me—while he sat in his office at a fast-paced New York law firm—for as long as it would take me to vomit madly, kneeling on the bathroom floor in our apartment sixty blocks away. A doctor had made an error and given me a medication that raised the blood level of my cyclosporine to near toxicity. At the moment I felt the nausea hit, I called Scott at the office and asked him if he would "stay with me" while I threw up; as much as he didn't want to listen to the violent heaving that would surely follow, he said yes. I told him that I was worried because of what I'd read in Columbia's transplant handbook, my survival bible: that vomiting and/or diarrhea can be very dangerous for transplant patients. What I didn't know, though, was that it was not the act of vomiting itself that posed a threat but rather the effects of fluid loss that could cause harm; and of course there was the risk of not being able to keep my immunosuppressive medicines in my stomach long enough for absorption. This important distinction would come to light only after Scott had spent longer than he thought he could possibly stand on the other end of my desperate and disgusting phone call. He proved himself to be a reticent but steadfast listener, cringing and turning his head away from the telephone receiver but hanging on the line to the very end, only to hear me cry out between heaves: "Are you still there? I need you to be there for me!"

"I'm right here. I'm not going anywhere." The voice of calm. The voice of infinite love.

Never let go . . . never let go. . . .

It was not until months after my distraught phone call, and after our wedding, that Scott told me he'd nearly thrown up himself while listening to my retching that day. By the time his truth came out, the whole episode of "Amy's vomit call" had turned into a bit of a joke, the kind of husband-wife ribbing that could be shared with friends and family for the sole purpose of eliciting comic relief. *Did I ever tell you about the day Amy called me out of a meeting so I could listen on the phone while she vomited for ten minutes? Yeah, my wife just hates to vomit. Yeah, really. Hates it even more than your wife does, don't kid yourself. And she won't do it alone. My wife likes to share her puking on the telephone.*

Ha, ha, ha.

How entirely devoid of humor were the truths Scott and I had come to know in our short time together. We had dated for just one year; been engaged for just one more. But, oh, the burdens we had withstood and the memories we carried. Joined, finally, at the altar—hand grasping hand, arm through arm, holding on for dear life in every sense possible—Scott and I were not a typical bride and groom beginning their journey into a life entwined. We had already journeyed far, into the depths of insidious illness and back out again. We had also come to know the flip side of the miracle: the torments of being saved. Together we'd lived both horrors and wonders, the kind of extremes that couples who have been married fifty years may never share and may be content to avoid.

And now tonight, my groom and I stood polished and seemingly perfect before a crowd of loving witnesses—a dazzling young couple about to set out into the world and become one. But Scott and I were certain even before taking our wedding vows that we were already one, otherwise we wouldn't have made it to this night. Our time together had already proven—without formalized promises of devotion, for better or worse—that while there was much that could have siphoned the air out of our love, there was even more that had somehow breathed life into it—and around it. There was a vital separation between our relationship and the illness that might otherwise have smothered it to death. Call it true love. Call it the work of an angel in Scott's body. Call it the grace of a grand plan of the universe.

I called it luck. On my wedding night, alive and well enough, I felt like the luckiest woman who'd ever fallen in love. All I had been hiding away on my walk down the aisle took on a new light as I saw it reflected in the eyes of my beloved. Every nightmare that had followed my diagnosis of cardiomyopathy, I now realized, could also be seen as a dream come true. At this moment, I was able to see my life as one of counterbalances, a combination that probably saved me more than once and made this wedding day possible. Set against the freakish illness that nearly killed me there was Scott's unwavering love. For every misstep made in my early diagnosis, later there were smart physicians and nurses in the right places at the right time. There was the unshakable optimism of my father and Beverly, which urged me on toward a wedding date I could only half believe in. And then there was the heart of a thirteen-year-old girl, a perfect match, that unfathomably had become my own—almost as if it had dropped out of the sky just for me.

Okay, I thought to myself as I came to the end of the satin carpeted aisle, *so maybe I am a heart-transplant patient. Maybe I am a sick girl who's been given an outrageously unlucky break.*

But at the same time, I glimpsed another side of my post-transplant life, bright and clear and shining beneath a white canopy. If what had befallen me and my poor body could only mean I was indeed unlucky, then surely I was the luckiest unlucky girl there ever was.

My father and I came to a stop beside Scott. We knew from the wedding rehearsal that this was the point where my father was supposed to lift a wisp of veil for a moment, lean down, and kiss me on the cheek. He did all this just as we had practiced. But then, in an unanticipated move, he bowed slightly toward Scott and asked, "May I interest you in a daughter?" This caused a chain reaction of laughter in the ballroom from front to back as guests repeated in whispers the wedding punch line that had not been entirely unexpected from my quipster father.

Scott joined in the laughter for a moment and then became solemn, grasping my father's hand in a firm handshake as if in final agreement: yes, he was infinitely, and most seriously interested in this very daughter. The deal at last finalized, my father disengaged his arm from mine so Scott could take his place beside me for the first time that night. Together, Scott and I continued up the few steps to the altar, leaving behind the teary-eyed funnyman who'd just given me away. At the moment we began to move forward, my father sprang up in the air and clicked his heels to the side in a rare showing of physical comedy. But really, he was not joking this time; my father was literally jumping for joy.

18

Later, during the cocktail hour, I basked in the glow of the healthy-bride illusion I'd carried with me down the aisle. Guests approached in frenzy, arms waving, joyous, eagerly on board with the spectacle they'd just seen on display at the ceremony. One of my father's cigar-smoking pals was among the first to set out after me, waddling enthusiastically to where I was stationed by the buffet table. Before reaching me, he called out, "Look at you, would ya! Beau-tee-ful girl! The picture of health, wouldn't you know!"

His wife caught up with him, stuffing the last bit of what looked like a mini crab cake into her mouth. Becoming suddenly weepy at close sight of me, she patted the corners of her eyes with her cocktail napkin. "It's all so . . . so . . . wonderful. This wedding. You. Here today. It's . . . it's. . . ."

Huge sobs.

"What she means to say is that we're both so happy for you—that you're all better now." The husband plucked the cigar from his mouth and pressed his mossy lips against my cheek.

I cringed. *He thinks I'm all better now!*

It felt as if this man had just congratulated me on doing exquisitely well with my monkey heart. How could he be so blind?

Because I'd set him up for it, that's how. I'd practically forced him—and everyone else in the room—to see me that way. I'd held myself strong and tall throughout my wedding march, even when I felt the wild denervated snapping of my heart midway down the aisle, which urged me to stop so the adrenaline could work itself out. But I'd continued on, smiling broadly. And when the wedding vows were read aloud—*in sickness and in health, till death do us part*—I held back tears of mixed emotion. I knew that Scott and I were beginning a life together that would contain more sickness than health, and that the way death could part us might be tragically premature.

For all the guests who wondered what could possibly make a terrific guy like Scott still want to marry me after such a life-altering surgery, I made sure to appear worthy of Scott's love and ongoing devotion, spending most of the evening in his arms on the dance floor, beaming my best smile and throwing my head back with carefree laughter. And for the many people in the ballroom who knew little or nothing about heart transplants—including those who would confuse the perilous implantation of artificial hearts (which barely kept their recipients alive in trial studies) with transplanted ones—I gave them a brief but directed lesson in transplant basics: bad heart gone, healthy human heart in, normal life restored.

But if the people who'd witnessed my veiled promenade down the aisle had come away with the sense that I was as healthy and normal as a bride could be, this only meant that I had managed to blur their vision. I'd simply succeeded in what I had set out to do when I took my first step onto the wedding carpet. But now the cocktail hour had arrived and a sense of regret was beginning to creep in.

I felt so misunderstood. Achingly invalidated. But isn't that what I'd asked for? Why should these people have known any better? Transplants had been portrayed to them in the media only in extremes—the high of the post-transplant patient who'd run a marathon, and the low of the one who died almost immediately after receiving an organ with a mismatched blood type. Even before I stepped through the ballroom doors, some of the guests had already assumed that transplant was an absolute cure: a complex but foolproof heart replacement. The guests sat back in their seats during the ceremony and laid self-serving eyes on what appeared to be living evidence of their viewpoint. Still, there were many others with the opposite view, held with equal conviction; this group had been expecting to see me make my way down the aisle gripping a walker or sitting in a wheelchair.

I sure set them straight, didn't I?

Yes, I did. And I would never forgive them for letting me do it.

Medicine time arrived as an especially annoying obligation that night. All through the wedding reception, I anticipated that at the stroke of ten I would have to break away from my own party and pop a syringe in my mouth. A dose of medicine was necessary every twelve hours; there was no playing around with the timing. If I didn't get immunosuppressives into my bloodstream at the appointed hour, I would have more to deal with than just a glittering horse-drawn carriage changed back into a pumpkin; I could actually wind up losing my new heart to rejection. So when the time came, I ran—or glided decorously—out the doors of the ballroom, down one elegant hallway and then another, on a secret journey to rendezvous with the coat-check girl who held my health in her hands. Earlier in the day, I'd given her a bottle of cyclosporine to keep safe for me, along with a small can of apple juice (a much-needed chaser for the sulferous taste of the liquid I would have to swallow). She opened the bottom half-door of the coatroom when she saw me coming down the hall. The expanse of my hoop skirt just barely squeezed through.

I looked around. There wasn't a table or other flat surface sufficient for laying out my medical paraphernalia. I would need my coatroom sergeant to help me, then, and quickly follow a series of direct orders. "Okay. I'll take these and you hold that." I reached out for the small glass bottle of cyclosporine and the nozzle-topped syringe, while parting with the apple juice. I pulled the plastic stopper out of the medicine bottle with my teeth and held it there until I'd filled the syringe up to the 400 ml line. "Okay, now hold this." I handed over the cyclosporine, followed by the cork that I'd just taken from my mouth. "And now give me that, please. Open it first, if you could."

She popped the top on the apple juice can. I stepped away so it wouldn't spray on my gown.

Squirt: a shot of nauseating bitterness beneath my tongue.

Slurp: an audible swig of juice to stave off the gag reflex.

Done. Ellen would have been proud. She'd taught me the fine points of this tricky cyclosporine/apple juice maneuver: the plastic stopper held between the teeth, the one-handed drawing up of medicine into the syringe, and the holding off of the final gulp until the apple juice was at the ready to sweeten the swallow.

A quick dash now, through the gilded hallways of the Pierre Hotel, and I would be back at my grand wedding, looking no worse for the wear, certainly, but feeling quite different than before my coatcheck rendezvous. Cyclosporine was poison to me, and soon it would be sweeping through my bloodstream, causing all kinds of side effects. In just a few minutes, nausea would take hold and rock my limbs with an unbearable case of land-borne seasickness; it would be a challenge for me to put a fork into a slice of my own wedding cake without retching. Then the shaking would turn more intense, finally driving me off the dance floor. There would also be a headache, the usual medicine-induced kind that always twisted my face into an inconsolable wince. If I weren't careful, this pain would surely rob me of the radiant smile I'd displayed so proudly from the moment Scott lifted the veil off my face for our wedding kiss.

Again, I would use my veil for cover, though not in the absolute sense (my wedding dresser had taken the veil from me after the ceremony). By quietly and gracefully fighting my way through side effects that could have ratted me out as being the sickened heart-transplant patient that I was, I would effectively reach out for my beautiful veil again and put it to good—if crafty—use. Instead of hiding myself beneath its generous draping, this time I would pull its blinding whiteness over the eyes of four hundred unsuspecting wedding guests. It was a sleight of hand, really—wedding style. The audience would see only what I wanted them to see: a crowd-pleasing illusion, a trick well done.

A heart transplant erased.

19

WHAT IS TEN YEARS TO A TWENTY-FIVE-YEAR-OLD WOMAN? MOST likely a long, busy, enjoyable time. It could very well encompass a career, marriage, a child or two, the beginnings of a few wrinkles around the eyes, maybe a small skin cancer nipped in the bud, the death of a favorite grandparent, three leased cars come and gone, a change in hairstyle or political party, a thirtieth birthday celebration, followed some slow-motion years later by a thirty-fifth, and then perhaps a quick look ahead toward a fortieth with easy disinterest: "Oh, forty—that's so far away." And, of course, it was far away—or at least would appear this way from the perspective of the young and trouble-free who've still got enough innocence left to believe they have forever on their side.

But I had lost my innocence.

As the horror of what happened to me settled in with the passing of time and became tinged with an increasingly philosophical viewpoint, I came to divide people into two categories: those who face serious illness early in life, and those who avoid medical tragedy straight into old age. At some point, it seemed, everyone would have their body stolen from them—and, with it, the ability to set themselves apart from medical misfortune. But timing is everything; the longer this loss can be delayed, the better. Being able to hold on to one's easy health, I came to believe, was the mark of true good fortune. The very lucky get hit later, simple as that.

I was twenty-five when Dr. Ganz offered me ten years—along with the surgery that would buy them for me: a heart transplant. Just moments before hearing this once-in-a-lifetime offer, I'd done the unthinkable and failed an electrophysiology test in the worst way, by flat-lining. But even this near-death experience had not robbed me of my youthful mindset—at least not yet. I was still just a woman for whom ten years could be perceived as a good long time. These years amounted to nearly half of my life so far. I flashed back quickly on a tumble of images and divided them into ten-year intervals—from birth to age ten, and from ten to twenty—and saw at once the tremendous changes in and around me that had been a natural part of the passage of time. I was amazed at all the living that could be stuffed into this small space. What couldn't I do in ten whole years? It was practically a lifetime. If I were to have this precious time with Scott, we would grow old together—into our midthirties, just imagine. I could finish law school, work as an attorney, live the New York City life I always wanted, see my friends marry off and my father and Beverly pass the sixty-five-year mark. I could learn a new instrument, a new language. Read a hundred books. Maybe even write one.

Yes, ten years sounded pretty good to me as I lay in a recovery room just minutes after slipping through death's fingertips. To be able to project myself up and out of this moment and into the future—a date that was far enough away to blur the reality of how close ten years really was—made Dr. Ganz's offer seem like a generous gift. It was a notion I could hold on to in the moment when I found myself grasping for something—anything—positive. It was hope. It was enough.

Until it wasn't anymore.

Time passed more quickly after my transplant than I'd anticipated. Perhaps this was because of the way I counted the years: one post-transplant year, two, three, and so on, until somewhere around seven years, when I redirected the count to be more future-focused—

death-focused, as it were. Year eight would become "two years left before I'm supposed to die," and year nine was the one-year warning for my impending demise. At ten, the whole counting system shifted into a borrowed-time scenario, where the years became eggshells that I would walk on with ever-decreasing confidence: I should have been dead one year ago; I should have been dead two years ago. . . .

Ten years was no longer a gift, it was a curse. With the squeaking by of each unlikely year, I felt more and more vulnerable. Reality was not my friend; data showed that transplant recipients like me were unique in how their likelihood of survival decreased as time went by. The "cure" that transplant patients receive (a donor organ and immunosuppression) actually lowers their chances of living disease-free over time. There is no point at which, statistically, a heart-transplant patient is on safer ground, because from the moment a donor heart begins to beat in a foreign chest, the immune processes of the body begin to destroy it. Since the day of my transplant, this very process had been happening inside of me. I knew it and sensed it, and my annual exams showed the beginnings of it—but at the same time I still had a strong sense that I was very much alive and way too young to die.

My mind did not reconcile well with the creeping awareness of a time-bomb heart. It left me with a blank, confused space between my thoughts and caused a disconnect between wishful thinking and reality. How could I be twenty-five—or twenty-six, or twenty-seven—and be so close to death? It didn't make sense. My mind pulled me toward the normal and ordinary for a woman in my age group—cute shoes, new lipstick colors, marriage, career choices—while my body tugged hard in the opposite direction, toward artery disease, rampant infections, medicines with side effects, and a life expectancy that had begun to seem rather optimistic, given the suffering and death that I saw around me in the transplant clinic waiting room. Like the puckered scar that ran down the center of my chest, there was a division within me I could not escape; I was part young woman, part sick girl. Neither part of me knew what to make of my split self—or my ever-shrinking ten years. People around me—friends, family, and even doctors—had some ideas of how to view myself. But as much as these good people might have wanted to understand, they could only see my life through their own, so their words would leave me as confused and frustrated as ever.

Only lonelier.

Long after my wedding night was over, the picture-perfect images I'd created during my walk down the aisle, out on the dance floor, and in front of the buffet table would become the enduring public illusion of what it was like to live in my body with a heart transplant. And I would feel forever compelled to keep it up somehow. In the name of appearances, I would spend my post-surgery years hiding away in a never-ending series of coat closets like the one I'd sought out at the Pierre, midway through my wedding celebration. Except for Scott, hardly anyone in my life had the opportunity to glimpse the jealousy, fear, and frustration inside of me; details of ugly things like heart biopsies, dead transplant friends, and sickening medicines were mine alone to know and keep quiet about. With sustained effort, I was able to create and enjoy everyone's false impression of my transplant life.

Then resentment set in. After a few years of trickery, I began to expect the people in my life to recognize in me the very things I'd fought so hard to hide. I came to rail against everyone I knew and loved for not seeing through my screen of normalcy—for not busting open the coat closet, grabbing hold of my oily bottle of cyclosporine, and demanding, "What *is* this stuff? Why do you have to take it? How sick does it make you feel?"

Instead, I got what I had asked for on my walk down the aisle: misunderstanding. Misunderstanding that hurt. Misunderstanding that ground away at me until I felt like the loneliest sick girl who ever lived a day with a heart that wasn't hers. Misunderstanding that took the form of a dangerously attenuated inner fuse that would ultimately short circuit a good deal of my patience, grace, and kindness.

Sometimes I'd lash out.

I once complained to Lynn, a close friend, that I'd just been diagnosed with another sinus infection—my eleventh in less than a year. Yet again, I'd been put on a twenty-one-day dose of heavy-duty antibiotics, and my sinus doctor admitted that he was beginning to run out of ideas. But Lynn, a cheery problem solver and highly educated suburban housewife, wasn't at all daunted; she had a terrific idea of her own—a well-informed layperson's medical solution. And she was going to share it, without the slightest hesitation or self-doubt, over tea and a piece of pound cake split down the middle.

"You've got to stop getting all these infections, and that's the bottom line," she said, beginning her usual step-by-step approach to unpleasantness that needed fixing. "You know what I think? I think you should do what the AIDS patients do. They have problems with low immunities, just like you, don't they? I read somewhere about these new drugs that help AIDS patients fight off infections by pumping their immune systems way up. If you just found out what the pills are and got your doctor to prescribe them for you, you wouldn't be so sick all the time."

Simple as that, huh? I didn't even try to hold back. "Yes, but I would be dead!"

Such unexpected unpleasantness at teatime. Lynn put her cup down and stared into it, intent on allowing the remaining rumbles of my thunder to dissipate before continuing on. "Don't be such a silly. Lots of people take these drugs; they're pretty common nowadays. And they don't make people die, that's for sure. These medicines actually save them."

"Well, I can promise you that I would die from them." Thunder was quickly giving way to an edgy nastiness. "A strong immune system would kill me real fast. My body would attack my heart. I'd be dead before my second dose of those AIDS pills. Yeah, they'd cure me of my sinus infections, all right. Cure me straight into my grave." Lynn shifted uncomfortably in her chair and raised her hand to the waiter, signaling for a check—*please*. A quick pang of regret told me maybe I shouldn't have been so hard on her, but I sure would have expected a dear friend like Lynn to understand more of the fundamentals of transplant immunosuppression, given that she'd seen me live by the sheer grace of them for so many years.

Then it occurred to me: perhaps Lynn would have been able to grasp *more* if I had hidden *less*.

I took a few calming breaths and continued. "You see, I take handfuls of pills every day just to keep my immune system *down*. If I wanted to lift my resistance to infection, all I would have to do is stop taking my medicine. I don't need more pills to strengthen my immune system—I need fewer ones. You see what I mean?"

She looked puzzled.

"It's like this. If I had more immune cells, white . . . blood . . . cells . . ."—I started to separate each word like an overwrought schoolteacher—"I would reject my heart. You know: rejection? The thing that can . . . kill me?"

The swipes had begun again.

"Sure, I know about rejection. A little bit anyway." Lynn pulled her wallet from her purse in anticipation of the arrival of the check and placed it down on the table next to mine. "And look, I was just trying to be helpful here. Sorry if I made a stupid suggestion. I guess I just misunderstood—your medicines, your transplant, the rejection thing. How it all works."

Yes, Lynn had misunderstood. And whose fault was that, really?

Mine.

Again, I found myself feeling the sting of the cover-up I'd been putting on for so long. Today Lynn felt it as well, and our friendship might not withstand the fallout. The consequences of hiding were quickly becoming too steep. Maybe for once it would be better if I just cleared away the fog, lifted the veil. I could open up to my good friend here and now, tell her all about the complexities and compromises of heart-transplant life. Then she would understand how the onset of another sinus infection could so easily become cause for intense despair and hopelessness; she would see the frustrating dead end that followed most of my post-transplant medical problems. Maybe the best thing to do, after all, was to be frank, honest, and understood rather than put on a show and be forever misconstrued.

Maybe.

The check still hadn't come. I tossed my wallet back into my bag and settled myself into a comfortable position that had some staying power; what I was about to say—or try to say—would carry me and Lynn through at least one more cup of tea. "Let me explain it to you, all right? Here is the problem with my medicines; really, it's kind of ironic if you think about it, but stay with me on this and I'll lay it all out for you. You see, I can't possibly take a drug that would increase my immune response, because then my transplanted heart—which my body recognizes as foreign—would be attacked."

But I'd already lost her. Lynn had begun to slouch down in her chair, not quite uninterested but not exactly eager to follow along either. I wrapped up the conversation with a shrug and a change of subject. My dear friend didn't seem to mind at all.

Soon the check arrived. We each set down a few dollars on the table and walked out of the café together.

Someone, please, hand me back my veil.

20

Dr. Davis, my transplant cardiologist, was among the first in a series of well-meaning people to grab hold of my post-transplant point of view and try to bend it, gently if crookedly. His efforts began one afternoon when I arrived at his office for an appointment. I dropped down into a chair on the other side of the desk and gave him a real scare.

"Can I have a baby?"

Dr. Davis wasn't ready for this question. It was only a few months after my wedding. The bounce in my step told him that married life was still aglow inside me with freshness and excitement; Dr. Davis couldn't imagine anything about my newlywed bliss that would be pressing down on me to have a baby right away. My post-transplant body was still fragile. A rejection episode —where my immune system would amass an army of white cells and lay siege to my new heart as if it were a dangerous invader— continued to be a real possibility for me at this point. So too was a transplant-related cancer, like lymphoma or an unstoppable melanoma.

Have a baby?

"No."

My eyes welled up. I let the tears fall.

Dr. Davis jumped into self-correction. "What I'm really telling you is *No, not yet.*"

"When, then?"

He pursed his lips whistle-tight. Dr. Davis was a slow-talking doctor who was in the habit of taking in at least one full breath of air—and then letting it out with the utmost control—before easing into a sentence. But he had already become used to receiving and deflecting my fastballs by this point in our relationship; why had this particular one rattled him so? It would take me several more months of trying out a variety of rapid fire questions before I came to the conclusion that it was only talk of babies, parenthood, and pregnancy that elicited an open emotional reaction from this aloof doctor of mine, a man whose hospital-wide reputation for coolness was entirely deserved. In time I would also learn what was at the core of his sensitivity to this particular subject matter: Dr. Davis had only recently become a father.

I was perplexed by the way he squirmed and sputtered in the wake of my question. He'd already taken the requisite breath—in and out, slow and measured—but still he was holding off anxiously, not yet comfortable with the answer that the sufficient passage of time was now forcing from his lips. "Well, ah—you're going back to law school . . . ah . . . soon, right? You won't want to have a baby until that's all done."

Dr. Davis was right. In just a few weeks I would return to NYU to complete my third year of studies. Better to delve into two hundred pages of complicated case law each night without having to tend to a crying baby at the same time. But law school wasn't going to last forever; if all went according to plan, I would finish up in just ten months.

Could I get pregnant right after graduation?

"We'll talk about it when the time comes."

I wanted to talk now.

Now was not an option for Dr. Davis; he'd already pushed his chair away from the desk and was beginning to stretch his extensive legs to stand.

"Whoa. . . . Wait a second, doctor, okay?"

Obviously it wasn't, but I continued anyway in a gust of chatter, squeezing as many words as I could into the five paces between my chair and his door.

"Can you just tell me before I go, please, whether heart-transplant women have babies? Can they have them, I mean? Do you have any patients who've gone through a pregnancy? Are the babies healthy? Do the transplant medicines harm them? Are there any statistics for—"

"When the time comes, we'll talk about it." His hand came down deliberately on the doorknob.

"All right, all right. But for now it would just be—well, um—helpful . . . if I could know whether there's a chance that I could have a—"

"When the time comes," he said, flat and final.

The door stood open to the hallway. Dr. Davis held it there with his hand, eager to usher me out. I began to move past him slowly, chin falling onto my chest, gathering up whatever courage I could in the final ten seconds that were left of his dwindling attention. My feet stopped midway through the door; I'd found my determination.

"I'm not going to let this disappear, you know. I am going to ask you about it again," I said, craning my neck to look way up into Dr. Davis's eyes with the most pulled-together, resolute expression I could muster, given my tearstained face and runny post-cry nose. But his eyes had already frozen over with professional distance; the baby softness had drained from them completely, leaving behind a no-nonsense sternness that made it all too clear that there was nothing about my pregnancy question that held any present-tense relevance. There was only the future. With just a few well-chosen words, a smirk of annoyance, and a door held open for me as a signal of finality, Dr. Davis had managed to move my sights ahead in time and cement them there. It was exactly what he intended to do.

There remained only seconds for me to give my final warning. "This baby thing is simply on hold, I promise you. I just have to finish law school—"

"Then go finish," he said.

It was the kick I needed, and Dr. Davis knew it. Acting on the knowledge that I had been a Phi Beta Kappa, magna cum laude, Dean's List kind of gal before my transplant and that a carrot of academic achievement dangled strategically in my future would be enough to keep me moving forward with intense focus, Dr. Davis was able to ensure two whole semesters of ideal psychological orientation for my post-transplant life. He tapped into my desire to succeed in law school and put aside my baby wishes for a convenient slice of time. As a result, I was likely to be happier, more productive, and less anxious in my immunosuppressed body and newly compromised life—if a bit manipulated. Any wool over my eyes would have been pulled there for my own good.

I returned, then, to law school with a decidedly narrow focus on academics. Scott took a job as an associate at the law firm where we first met, and I kept my head buried in massive textbooks and law journals. I would kiss Scott as he left for work each morning; I'd greet him each evening with a home-cooked dinner. For the long hours in between, I was an NYU law school student with a sense of urgency that bordered on vengeance; damn it, I would get through the day—the month, the semester, the year—no matter what. I raced through the remainder of law school in spite of my body, with a bottle of cyclosporine tucked in my left coat pocket and a small can of apple juice stuffed into my right—well prepared, of course, for my 10 A.M. trip to the bathroom, where I'd hide in a stall, squirt medicine into my mouth, and then hurry off to class.

Sometimes illness would slow me down or keep me away from school, landing me in the hospital for a few days or even a week; other times I'd be held back by my denervated heart, which made it hard to stand beside my desk—as was required—to answer a professor's pointed question in front of the class. But I was intent on forging forward and also on hiding my transplant wherever possible. April rolled around and I congratulated myself, not only for having made it to my final set of exams but also for not having allowed any of my classmates to glimpse my cyclosporine bottle even once.

Graduation arrived before I knew it and I found myself back in Dr. Davis's office; I was a Juris Doctor ready for my pregnancy talk.

"I graduated last week. Can I have a baby?"

It was eleven months after I'd first raised the issue. Two years after my surgery, one year after my wedding. The day had arrived when I could hold my head high, pose my question to Dr. Davis for the second time, and get an answer.

Or had it?

"Pass the bar exam first, why don't you," he said. "We'll talk after that."

The exam was only two months away. It was critical to my legal career. The best thing for me would be to put up with two more months of waiting.

I went on to pass the bar exam, which to me seemed like a giant step toward pregnancy more than anything else. But for my friends and family, the achievement was in itself a cause for celebration. On the surface, passing the bar was purely good news to them, insofar as they could compare their own completion of graduate school exams and requirements to mine. Everyone thought they knew what it took to pass. They'd been there themselves, in one form or another. It was assumed, then, that there was an understanding between us, a commonality. We saw the taking and passing of exams in the same way.

But really, we didn't at all. What my friends did not know was that I bled during the bar exam, right through my pants and onto the faux wood seat of my chair. Not just a little blood, a sopping pool of it. From the get-go, my transplant medicines had caused terrible problems with my period, and I would bleed from week to week instead of month to month, a gush out of nowhere, sometimes dangerously heavy. I had begun the bar exam without any hint of blood but ended it six hours later with pants stained and soaked through, red-purple, right down the backs of both thighs.

When I felt the first unmistakable sense of what was about to flow from me, I put my pencil down beside my answer sheet and took a precious moment of testing time to close my eyes and make a silent vow: *I will finish this exam even if I bleed to death.* When I'd finally filled in the last answer bubble, I wrapped my NYU Law sweatshirt around my waist, dabbed the chair with some tissues from my purse, and walked to the subway, blood-wet denim clinging to my legs. Before long, Scott and I were on our way to the hospital. It took two full bags of donated blood—a transfusion—to replace what I'd lost in the span of a few hours.

But I'd passed the bar exam all right. That's what my friends saw and understood. And so they rejoiced—as did my family and even my doctors. But their enthusiastic pats on the back and cascades of congratulations were just like the suggestions they'd made about how I might best navigate my post-transplant life; all of them seemed naïvely optimistic.

I went back to Dr. Davis again, this time with more confidence than ever. "I passed. Now I can have a baby, right?"

"Why don't you go practice law for a while? Be an attorney; it's what you've wanted to do all these years, isn't it? After that, we'll see." Once again, it wasn't exactly a *no* but rather another fine attempt to reorient my perspective toward my career—still delivered in that cheery, encouraging way. This time, though, it didn't work.

Because there was no such thing as "after that." My job as an attorney didn't have a natural ending point. It was simply a corporate law position—for as long as I wanted it. There was no longer a moment of achievement for me to look forward to. No future point in time where I could again approach Dr. Davis and say, "I've done as you asked. Can we talk about a baby now?" From now on, the answer to that question would always have to be "No, not yet." My future was missing a goal.

I began tumbling in dizzying somersaults of unspecified time and purpose. When I turned right side up, on my feet again after clearing my mind of the shifts in perspective that had been pushed on me since my transplant (*just keep focusing on your wedding date,* Dr. Davis had insisted, *finish law school . . . pass the bar . . . work as an attorney*), I found myself floundering, with a now eight-year life expectancy staring me in the face.

I suddenly had endless questions for my doctor. The kind that would have—and perhaps should have—weighed more heavily on me over the years that had passed since my transplant. Questions like "Are my medicines killing me even as they're keeping me alive?" and "Will there come a point in this body when I won't be a sick girl anymore?" And then of course there was the most soul-wrenching question of all: "How am I supposed to wrap my mind around this life expectancy?" The floodgates had been opened and all illusions washed away. I was left only with the ugly bare bones of my reality. Dr. Davis's perspective game had played itself out.

It was a game that had to end badly, and it did.

There in the silence, in the stillness that came after my realization that the answer would always be *No, not now,* I understood I wasn't going to have a baby after all.

And now I only had eight years left to live—at best.

Eight years! How could that be?

I was only twenty-seven.

21

IT TOOK AWHILE AFTER MY TRANSPLANT TO HEAR THE TICKING CLOCK of my new heart, but once I did, the sound became unbearably loud. No one around me would hear it the same way I did. As visible as the signs were—hospitalizations, clinic visits, heart biopsies, illnesses, and infections—it seemed that everyone preferred to pay attention to other things about me.

"You always make the best salad!" they'd rave.

Tick-tock, tick-tock.

"Your hair looks great! Did you do something different?"

Tick-tock, tick-tock.

"Scotty really outdid himself this time. Would you look at those beautiful earrings!"

Tick-tock, tick-tock.

The truth was, I'd been sick when I made that salad, so weak I had to sit down at my kitchen table three times before I even got around to chopping the tomatoes. And yes, I'd had a great haircut just last week, but I'd made the mistake of taking my medicine just before my shampoo, and by the time the scissors made the first snip I was fighting back the strong urge to throw up in my lap. The earrings too were pure sparkle at first glance, but they came with an unspoken burden as well: the thought that I might not be able to wear them enough times to make Scott's purchase worth it.

It was thoughts like these—along with the *tick-tock* that turned into a wailing siren as the years passed—that finally landed me in a therapist's office. I needed to make sense of things.

Dr. Fisher, the therapist I chose for this task, wasted no time in summing up the answer to my predicament; he ended one of our early sessions by telling me, "Suffering is suffering."

This clincher was supposed to make me feel better about my heart transplant and my limited life expectancy?

Dr. Fisher threw up his hands in a take-it-or-leave-it gesture, resting his case for the day. He'd managed to take everything I'd poured out to him and turn it into a useless three-word platitude.

The following week, I nearly plugged my ears with my fingers when I recognized that, again, Dr. Fisher was searching for a situation comparable to mine—one that involved a young woman who'd suffered an illness that was more common than mine but just as challenging. When it became apparent that he couldn't find a useful parallel, Dr. Fisher tried to hit his point home anyway. "One person's stubbed toe . . ." he said, and then paused midsentence to see whether I would finish his thought with something I'd learned during one of our sessions (I wouldn't), ". . . is another person's heart transplant."

I told him I didn't think so. "They cut my heart out with a knife. My heart! It doesn't make any sense."

"Sure it does. Just look at the biology of your illness. It's understandable that a virus might attack and destroy part of the body. And replacing your heart with one that works better? May I propose to you—it might be looked at as changing a piece of plumbing. A simple pump standing in for the one that stopped working."

I told him no, he might not propose to me something so completely ridiculous. Dr. Fisher took this as evidence that I actually preferred suffering to rearranging my perspective in a helpful way, and to him this was even more ridiculous.

But my experience with Dr. Davis and the ongoing baby question had taught me that playing with perspective can be a dangerous business.

Not as dangerous as unnecessary suffering, Dr. Fisher argued. If I insisted on continuing to view my transplant in the same old way, I would suffer more that I had to. Wasn't that a silly way to live?

If only I would be a compliant patient and spin my head around a few times so I could view my pre-transplant illness as having been a normal everyday occurrence. Dr. Fisher offered up one final pearl of wisdom in this regard: "Life is short, it's full of shit, and then you die," he said. "Shit happens."

Not this kind of shit.

"Of course it makes sense scientifically," I told him, "but not realistically. Cancer happens. Car accidents. Even a paralyzing dive into shallow water happens. But what happened to me doesn't happen. Twenty-five-year-olds don't get their hearts cut out."

"Oh, but they do, you see. You did."

"That's not what I meant."

"But it's what you said, isn't it? You said that what happened to you doesn't happen. But as you see, it did."

I felt I'd just followed Alice down the rabbit hole.

"It's all how you look at it, Amy. Your perceptions are everything. It's not what happens to us that matters, but how we view it."

And shall we have some tea, O Mad Hatter?

I would show him his clichés were no match for this sick girl's reality. "Check out my view, why don't you? I'm going into the hospital for my annual exam next week, a heart biopsy and an angiogram. It's year eight. I was given ten. How am I supposed to view that?"

"Here's how. You are going to be the miracle that lives twenty years. Thirty years. Forty. You simply think about it this way. You see?"

"You're a fool."

"A fool who doesn't want to suffer."

"A fool who lives in la-la land."

"Perhaps, but I'll suffer less while I'm there. Heh, heh!"

Dr. Fisher perched on the edge of his leather recliner, leaning in toward me for the grand finale. "May I propose to you . . ."

Oh, no, not again. I began to search through my handbag for my date book, purposely self-distracted.

This only made his eyes bug out. "May I propose to you . . . that anything you face in life has no reality in and of itself. It only exists as you choose to see it."

I paused at the door for a moment. *Could I actually think this way and believe it?*

Was it possible that I—a young woman who'd once set out optimistically in the face of a heart virus, but who wound up with defibrillator paddle burns and a heart transplant—could take on the attitude of someone whose cheerful outlook had never been pounded down by near death?

If only I could. . . .

I told Dr. Fisher I'd give it some thought. What I didn't tell him, though, was that I would do my thinking transplant style: flat on my back, my hair tucked away inside a surgery cap, with one catheter lodged in my neck and another one stuck into an artery in my groin. I revisited Dr. Fisher's therapeutic suggestions a few days later—on the table at my annual exam.

22

SCOTT'S LOVE ALWAYS SEEMED TO SWELL UP AND SHOW ITS TRUE depth and expanse right around the time of my annual exam. But really, his affection and devotion were close to bursting all year long. His constancy amazed me.

Even eight years after my transplant, Scott looked at me with the same adoring eyes and the same sparkle emanating from his sweet soul. I'd seen this glow first when we were law associates together. But I was older now—and not as pretty as I would have been had illness not stolen away my loveliness too soon. The many years of post-transplant medications and illnesses had taken their toll, aging me more quickly than nature otherwise would have. And Scott had seen so much of me over these years—much too much, really. He'd carried my bedpans long before we were even engaged to be married. He'd run his fingers across the thick dark hair that grew on my back and chest due to the high doses of medication in the first few years after my transplant, even assuring me that he liked my "furriness." Scott had pretended not to notice the prednisone-induced potbelly that hung on after my surgery for longer than both of us would have liked. He cleaned up my vomit—many times. He accompanied me to emergency rooms. He sacrificed. He withstood.

And time after time, year after year, Scott watched as each of his friends married gorgeous, unblemished, healthy, trouble-free women, and he didn't flinch.

At least he never let me see him do it.

I couldn't help but marvel from time to time that Scott had married me. He'd taken on all the ugliness of illness in loving stride, never wavering in his devotion and never complaining. He had made a conscious choice to allow his healthy, carefree life to take on my sick, difficult one, and feeling love with a depth that left me awestruck—just the way it had when I glimpsed his shining figure standing in the doorway of my hospital room. This was a man who loved me to the core, who thought I was desirable, adorable, and sexy whether I was sick or well, old or young, near death or battling to stay far from it. It didn't matter whether I was in a hospital gown, an old pair of pajamas, or even naked with a thick telltale scar running down the center of my chest; Scott would behold me like some kind of a bombshell. He'd give me the eye, shake his head a couple of times, and tell me, "You are stunning," and in saying this it was he who would stun me. I could not have given Scott more ugliness, and yet he still managed to find my points of beauty.

Because love was his compass.

But it was not a compass that could provide all the direction I needed in my transplant life. Scott's love could only get me so far. I had hoped Dr. Fisher could take me the rest of the way. But on the eve of my eighth annual exam I felt the heavy, tiring sense of how much navigation I would still have to do on my own.

Scott pulled *The New York Times* out of his briefcase and flashed me a knowing smile. "Let's do it now," he said.

I understood exactly what he meant: the crossword puzzle. The day's *New York Times* crossword was a vital part of a shared superstition that Scott and I couldn't help but carry along with us into the waiting room of the angiogram suite each post-transplant year. The possibility of the crossword's magical powers—however unlikely—was enough to compel us to complete as much of the day's puzzle as possible, preferably huddled together on the small couch in the far corner of the room, taking turns filling in the blanks with the same pen: one answer for me, one for him. This silly but irresistible ritual would presumably work some kind of magic to ensure that the results of my annual exam would be just as good as they had been in previous years and the doctors would see only a small amount of transplant-related disease in my arteries, insignificant and nonprogressing.

Scott and I had almost always gotten through whole puzzles in the past before the angiogram nurse, Mary, arrived to escort me back to the dressing room. But today we'd barely managed to finish the upper left corner of the grid; she came out to fetch me earlier than usual. Kindly Mary couldn't possibly have guessed that her premature arrival might alter the outcome of my exam. But Scott and I knew; our eyes locked in mutual concern when we heard her voice ring clear across the waiting room a full ten minutes before my scheduled appointment time.

"You can come on back now, Amy," she called out from the door, singsong, more like the shampoo girl at my haircutting salon than a nurse at a cardiac center. "We're ready for you!"

But I wasn't ready for them. With only the upper left corner of the crossword boxes completed—half in Scott's semiscript scribble and half in my tidy capital letters—how could I be sure the puzzle gods would save me today?

"Scotty." I grabbed his hand so tightly that he winced and pulled away, as if from electric shock.

"Ouch! Hey!"

"Sorry, honey! Oh, I'm so sorry!"

Damn, I'd gone and done it again—squeezed Scott's hand with the kind of intensity that would crush the edge of his wedding band right into that tender bony spot halfway down his middle finger. He hated when I did this.

We were not going to get to finish the crossword puzzle this year. But I still had my lucky blue stretch pants, thank goodness. Scott didn't recognize at first that these pants, like our puzzle ritual, were infused with power, though he'd noticed today that I was wearing them—again.

"Didn't you wear those last year?" he asked.

I played it equally cool. "I guess so, I don't know. They're sort of . . . comfortable."

"Mmm."

He knew. Even without my telling him, Scott understood that I held tight to a few good-luck charms of my own—ones I didn't care to share. And I'm sure he too had a couple of secret talismans.

"Amy, yoo-hoo over there! Ya ready?" Mary continued to hold the door wide open for me with a straight strong arm and an unrelenting grin.

Just as in other years, I was at once overwhelmed by a feeling that I was a marked animal being coaxed into a deadly trap. Instinct forced me to recoil. A premonition came to mind in screaming hues—sickening reds, wretched gray blacks, screaming oranges—all brought into the moment by the enduring memory of too many terrible forays into the wilds of cardiac testing rooms. Yes, blood was going to flow today, my blood. And a life was going to be judged by external, uncontrollable powers.

My life.

"I don't want to go in there, Scotty. I don't want to do this again. They might tell me I'm dying. It could be all over."

"You're going to be fine."

"I might never see you again. I could die on the table. These exams have risks, you know."

"Don't be silly."

"It could happen. . . ."

Scott shut his eyes tight for a moment and shook the sudden pins and needles from the back of his neck. "Come on, now. It's time. I'll see you when it's all done. Go on. Mary's waiting."

"Scotty." One last tearful gaze and I broke away from him, touch by touch—forehead, arm, hand, fingers. The pen we'd shared dropped to the floor as I stood up; Scott didn't bother to get it. He was holding my eyes.

"I love you so much, Amy." He bit down on his lip. I thought he might cry, but no; Scott would not allow this. Not in front of me. One of us had to pretend that this wasn't such a big deal.

I picked up the pen from the floor and held it out to him. "In case you want to finish the puzzle without me," I said.

"No. Can't do it without you." That was the superstition talking. Scott brought my hand up to his lips and mumbled between my fingers in a desperate whisper, "Can't do the puzzle without you . . . can't do anything without you. You know that. So go on in there and be strong. Do what you have to do. And then you come back to me, okay? I'll save the puzzle for us. We'll finish it together, later, all right?"

I began to weep. "Guess so. Love you."

Scott watched me walk to the door. "Love you!" he called out, as Mary swung her arm around my shoulder and led me into the angiogram suite. The weighty radiation-proof door closed behind us with a loud, lonely click that shut out Scott and all his love for the next two hours.

The sign on the door read CATHETERIZATION LAB: AUTHORIZED PERSONNEL ONLY.

I would never know what it was like for Scott to be held prisoner in that waiting room; he would never know what I faced in the belly of the cath lab. From the moment I left Scott behind, we each entered our private and distinct world, the ugly details of which we kept to ourselves. When it came to this annual exam, Scott and I were in silent solemn agreement that this was one of those times in a marriage—in a love, in a shared life—when it was preferable to be left a little in the dark.

Did Scott drop his forehead into his hands and hold it there, eyes closed tight, long after I'd disappeared behind the cath lab door? Did I break down in the dressing room—burying my face in the stretch pants I'd just taken off—murmuring, "I don't want to do this anymore . . . I don't want to do this anymore. . . ."

We would never say.

"Deep breath in now, Amy. We're going to take some pictures."

Soon I would know whether this was the year that untreatable transplant artery disease (or vasculopathy, as the doctors called it) had finally made its way into my heart and irrevocably damaged its blood-carrying arteries. All transplant patients get hit with it sooner or later, most of them within the first five years post-transplant. Vasculopathy was known well by patients to be the most serious and likely threat against them, and it is also the sneakiest; in most cases the disease hits hard, fast, and symptom free. Transplant patients are not likely to feel the signs and symptoms of clogged arteries, such as chest pain, since their new hearts are not attached to their central nervous systems. So it is entirely possible to spend the whole year between annual exams assuming that your heart is fine—you're feeling well enough, climbing stairs okay, riding a bike without too much trouble—but then when you get to the angiogram table—a terrible surprise: you've got widespread artery disease and need another heart transplant. Fast. You've been dying for months but didn't know it; your new heart tricked you, giving you a false sense of beating the odds.

Maybe that would be me on the table this year.

I felt the doctor's pointer finger tapping deliberately on the top of my right thigh; this was a signal to me that he was about to shoot the contrast dye into the artery plug that he'd just inserted into my groin. And here it was now: the telltale warm flush rising up through my abdomen, chest, neck, and face and back down again, the full length of my legs, all the way to my toes. I was now filled with dye. The camera started to whir, and there on the screen above the exam table I could see today's first picture of my arteries. There was a pause in the action as the doctors and nurses took a long hard look.

Silence.

There wouldn't be a better time than now for me to try out Dr. Fisher's suggestion. He'd insisted I could choose to see this exam and all its subparts any way I wished; the angiogram could be a neutral nonevent, if only I would set out to spare myself psychic pain. I could also choose to see my body in a way that would cause me less suffering; no good could come from doubting my longevity, no matter what the statistics said.

Okay, here goes: my body is strong and my heart is fine. I'm going to be the lucky transplant patient who never gets hit with artery disease. In fact, I expect that any minute now the doctor is going to call out, *Miracle! This girl is a miracle!* Aw, these angiograms aren't nearly as torturous as I thought—they're not bad at all, actually. It really depends on how you look at it. . . .

"I feel dizzy." It came over me suddenly. I thought the doctor should know.

No answer.

"I said I feel dizzy!"

The doctor turned his head toward a nurse and said something in an urgent mumble that I could not decipher, except for the final word: *stat.*

I froze: it was going to be the flat-line exam table all over again, wasn't it? Sudden dizziness, tense doctors talking low and muted, nurses following orders, *stat;* one last look at the world around me and then there would be no world around me at all. No me at all. It looked like my transplanted heart was about to do me in, just like my own heart had done me in eight years earlier.

But not just yet. As far as I could tell, I was still alive. No blackness. No nothingness. I worked to free my arm from the restraint one of the nurses had fashioned out of an edge of linen, and then I slid my hand up and out of the sterile draping so that I could pull the plastic all the way off my face. No one seemed to notice.

I cried out into the open air, "What's going on!"

The spiking lines on the EKG monitor got more attention than my shouting did. The doctor kept his eyes glued to the screen for a few more silent moments. Then he blinked once and spit out a prefab answer like some kind of programmed doctor robot. "Your heart is in spasm. We've given you something. To make it stop."

"Spasm? What! How?"

"It happens. Sometimes."

"Happens why?"

"I don't know."

"How could you not know? You're a cardiologist! You do angiograms all day long!"

"Yes."

"And there's nothing more you can tell me?"

"We've already given you something. To counter it. Now we watch. And wait." He nodded toward the EKG monitor.

I followed his glance over to the screen. The crazy up-and-down lines looked far from the "transplant normal" I'd come to recognize on printouts of my periodic EKGs. Something was wrong, and I still had the dizziness to prove it.

"Look, hey, um, somebody . . . please . . . I'm really scared here. Could one of you just . . . I need someone to . . . hold my hand . . . maybe?" My teeth had become chattering castanets, but I went on, clenching my jaw so I could continue my call for help. "Someone? Someone, please!"

No one. Sorry.

There were no less than six white-coated bodies in that cath lab—twelve warm comforting hands protruding from their sleeves. Yet I was left without a hand to hold. I was alone.

I was just a heart, beating ominously. Again.

The doctor let out a long loud deep breath, like air from a party balloon. I turned my head and saw him nod some kind of all-clear, and the nurses moved away from the table, back to their more typical duties. The spasm had finally subsided. This exam would now proceed on its way without further delay.

"Looks like we're going to be together for a bit longer than usual today. I'd like to take some extra pictures, just to be safe. Hope you can put up with me for another few minutes," the doctor said, the flow of his voice humming once again. "With the coming and going of that spasm, we weren't able to see your arteries too well. We couldn't tell what was disease and what was just spasm."

The mention of the word *disease* triggered Dr. Fisher in my head—how he himself might have reacted to it: *Oh, silly cardiologist, you're not going to find any disease! I'm the miracle patient, don't you know? I'm going to live thirty years.*

Like hell I am.

In all the annual exams leading up to this one, I had been afraid only of what the angiogram pictures might reveal. But now I had a new fear—one I'd never considered, never picked up from a conversation in the transplant waiting room, never even heard Ellen mention. From now on I would fear not just what the angiogram would reveal but the exam itself and all the risks I'd signed away so glibly on the pre-op consent form. *Spasm* was printed halfway down the page, I remembered. So was *heart attack* and *stroke*. I'd never believed these would happen to me. Now I knew they could.

"I heard from the doctor already—great news! You got some great news today!" A jubilant Scott was already waiting for me in the recovery area when the nurse rolled me in on a stretcher. He kissed me on the forehead, all smiles.

I started to tell him that my heart did "some funny stuff" during the exam and I'd been "kind of scared."

"Yeah?" He was feeling playful, still high on the good report he'd just heard, only half listening.

"They gave me something for it. After a bit, everything settled down."

"Oh, that's good. The doctor told me the pictures look fine. You've got beautiful arteries, my dear."

I'm a miracle, right? A miracle that could have died on the table today, if you really want to know.

But Scott didn't want to know. He shouldn't have to know.

"Hand me that bag, would you? The one with the muffin in it." I was hungry for some breakfast.

Scott broke into a wide grin and placed a fat blueberry muffin in my lap, along with a napkin. The day's rituals had finally come full circle, the post-exam muffin being the last of them. And they'd all worked their good magic, it seemed.

Scott moved his chair alongside me and put his elbows on the edge of my hospital bed. Just as I plucked off the first bite of crumb topping with my front teeth and rolled it onto my tongue, he reached one hand down into his briefcase and pulled out the folded crossword puzzle, still only one quarter completed.

"Let's do it," he said.

So we did.

The following week, I returned to Dr. Fisher with a story to tell.

"Please now, concentrate," I told him. "Imagine yourself on an exam table. There's a plastic sheet draped over your body from head to toe. . . ."

I asked him to imagine that he was about to have an invasive cardiac procedure, a test that would act as a sort of diagnostic crystal ball, calling forth images in quick vivid X-ray flashes that would reveal the future of his heart. Whether he might die soon. Whether he was dying already.

"You can't see anything or anyone. You can only hear and feel—the sound of your own breathing, the gallop of your heart. The doctors above you speak in muted tones that sound increasingly anxious. Suddenly you're dizzy. Gasping. No, sir, it doesn't look like you're going to make it through this exam. You're never going to get up off this table, are you? And there's no one there to hear your good-bye. Don't think for a minute that some cockamamie perspective is going to help you out now; the last few minutes of a failing heart don't give a crap about how you choose to see it. Death will squeeze until there's nothing left of you and your flimsy mind games."

He blanched.

One of his hands went up like a shot, covering his eyes, while the other waved me away with frenetic outward sweeps into the air. "Oh, no, no. I don't like to think about my own death. When I do, it freaks me out."

Then Dr. Fisher pulled out his undaunted mind-over-matter perspective and held it in front of him like a shield, as reassuring and self-protecting as he willed it to be.

"I'm going to live forever," he said.

Well, good for him.

23

In September of 1996, a miracle came my way. I put my corporate law job aside forever and welcomed this unexpected wonder into my life. It launched me on a hot-air balloon ride, up, up, and away from my usual self, so that for the first time in many years it was possible to experience a bit of unadulterated post-transplant enchantment.

My miracle was a baby.

I became a mother. Scott became a father. Our son was the miracle.

The cardiomyopathy specialist I'd seen years earlier in Boston—the one who'd rattled off a list of things I would never be able to do in my life, like climb stairs or play sports—had told me I would never have a baby. Even after my transplant, the baby news was not good. But no doctor ever told me I could not be a *mother*. I didn't have to carry a baby in order to love and raise one. This vital point would remain unmentioned by two cardiologists who could not see beyond the scientific and biological mechanics of parenthood.

"I'm worried about the effects of a cyclosporine carrier on a fetus," Dr. Davis told me, text book recitation style, after years of caginess and backpedaling.

I was a cyclosporine carrier. The drugs I took to keep me alive could harm my unborn child. Clarity rained down on me.

I wanted to be a mommy. I wanted to have a healthy baby.

In this thunderbolt moment, I felt like Dorothy at long last in the Emerald City, listening to the highfalutin argot of the wise but diminished Wizard of Oz. At journey's end, I opened my mind and realized, as young Dorothy did, that I'd always had the power to do what I wanted; I'd had it within me all along. I'd had to embark on a four-year walk-and-talk down the yellow brick road with Dr. Davis just to come home again to what had always been there for me to discover: I could still be the mother I wanted to be without playing the role of "carrier."

And Scott could be a father. The thought of parenthood was as much a joy for him as it was for me, and now with adoption in mind, what had seemed impossible for a heart-transplant couple was actually within our grasp. But there were still complications. Only two years remained of my life expectancy: would this mean our child might lose his mother before entering preschool? Scott gave a lot of thought to this question as the prospect of fatherhood became more real and concrete. He knew I might die. I knew it too. But we never talked about it, not until Casey grew to the age where my ten-year life expectancy had safely proved itself to be an underestimation. Only then did Scott tell me in a poignant moment, "I went into this adoption knowing I would probably wind up as a single parent before too long."

But, he said, he was sure our child would grow up in a home filled with love, for however many years I was alive and then beyond them. Scott was secure in his own vast capacity for caring and nurturing; this child of ours would be adored forever. And Scott and I would have had some time together as parents.

Precious time.

On one Indian summer day in the early fall, the baby we'd yearned for was born. Beautiful Casey: restorer of wonder and awe, maker of dreams come true: seven and a half pounds of wiggling, gurgling, bottle-sucking inspiration. It was this tiny swaddled body nestled in the crook of my elbow that would make me think again about the words spoken to me by a cowardly psychotherapist: *I'm going to live forever.* Even if this was nonsense, I was going to try like hell to make it real—if only for the sake of this baby boy.

Becoming a mom can do that to a woman. Like everyone else, I'd read real-life stories about mothers who'd lifted off the equivalent of a bulldozer pinning down their children. I too would be a mother called to action by a perceived threat to my child; in this case the threat was made against *my* life, the fight was for it—against the odds. From the first time I held little Casey in my arms, I determined to be part of my son's life for as long as possible. Or even for longer than possible. Please, I begged the great mother-strength that hums softly throughout the universe, let me live longer.

I was a mommy now. Mommies have to be there for their children. I knew what it was like to grow up with a mother who was absent even when she sat beside me at the dinner table, saliva dripping from her flaccid Johnnie Walker–numbed lips. My mother had been an obligatory carrier, a sufficiently cooperative presence for the time I grew within her, but soon after I was born she disappeared into a red labeled liquor bottle. That I might some day disappear from Casey—that my death might rob him of his mother the way alcohol had robbed me of mine—would turn me instantly busy with a diaper change or a frenetic round or two of "Row, Row, Row Your Boat." I was his life source. This baby boy needed me—for fresh diapers, for soothing songs, for food, and for patient, loving attention when he cried out in the middle of the night. Adoption did not change the mother I would be to my son, just as pregnancy had not changed the mother that mine had been to me. At 4 A.M., as I lay on the floor beside a bassinette, ever-ready with a newly sterilized pacifier in my hand, I knew there was no escaping the demands of motherhood; certainly not with a scotch on the rocks, and—if I had my way—not even in death. When Casey's hungry wail pierced the silence, I would jump from supine semislumber to loving attentiveness with the agility of an acrobat. And there, in the yellow glow of a little ducky night-light, I felt less like a sick girl than I had for as far back as I could remember.

My friend Ellen had told me there was something about being a mommy that could smooth out the sharp edges of a heart-transplant life and make a woman forget herself. Once, when Ellen and I were talking about the botched heart biopsy that explained the blood-stained bandage on her neck, she drifted into a faraway grin because her daughter had suddenly come to mind. She stopped the medical story and told me about Katie's costume for Halloween, how she'd made it for her this year and how it had come out terribly lopsided. "Wow, Mom," Katie had said to her, once contorted into the crooked jumpsuit, "you made it look even spookier!"

Some kind of terrific kid, huh?

What was a bloody post-biopsy neck when there was an angel child at home? Motherhood allowed Ellen to see beyond the stained bandages of her heart-transplant life. She made it plain to everyone she knew that her greatest happiness resided in her mommy moments—like when she made a peanut-butter-and-jelly sandwich and cut off the crusts. Standing in the kitchen with a smiley-face paper plate on the counter before her, there was nothing in Ellen's world but two slices of bread, some filling, and a hungry little girl.

Even before I became a mother myself, I would come to see the power of motherhood at work in Ellen—and also in another young heart-transplant patient. There were not many of us at Columbia, so we were easy to spot in the clinic waiting room. I approached Marissa because I'd been told about a woman who'd given birth to a baby after undergoing a heart transplant; the description seemed to fit.

"You must be Marissa," I said.

"Why must I be?"

"Well, I don't see a lot of young women here at the clinic. And I've been told that now there's another young heart transplant patient, named Marissa."

"You think there aren't a lot of young women in this place?"

"Oh, I really can't tell for sure. I usually put these on when I'm here anyway." I pointed to the small headphones that lay next to the Walkman in my lap. "I guess I don't pay a lot of attention to the crowd. But you are Marissa, aren't you?"

She nodded and stuffed two sticks of gum into her mouth, one after the other.

"Well, great. Because I've thought a lot about getting pregnant. And I've heard that you had a baby after your transplant."

"Yeah, and?" she said.

"Well, wow, good for you!"

"What do you mean?"

Marissa clacked her gum loud and angry. Her nostrils flared.

"Don't mind me. Maybe I'm just a big worrier—at heart. No pun intended." She didn't laugh. "Anyway, Dr. Davis got all weird when I asked him about having a baby. How 'bout you?" I assumed that Marissa and I had Dr. Davis in common.

"Davis isn't my doctor. I go to the other guy." *Clack*. Small bubble. *Clack*. "He told me just to do what I want."

"Of course he did."

And that's what we'd all done, wasn't it? One way or another, Ellen, Marissa, and I—we'd each done what we wanted. Ellen wanted to carry and love her daughter to the point where it overshadowed her three transplants and the grim likelihood of a fourth. Marissa too wanted to get pregnant and have a baby, and she refused to see her transplant as a good reason not to. And I wanted to be alive—for myself, for Scotty, and now for my son—for longer than my life expectancy was likely to allow; I would fight to lift my ten-year sentence the way I would a bulldozer crushing Casey's legs. By becoming mothers, all three of our heart transplants became lighter loads to carry. More than a beloved hobby, a career, or even a husband, it was motherhood that brought us back to ourselves.

I savored Casey's baby and toddler years, hoping I could slow them with vigilant, loving attention to every wonderful detail. But there was no holding on to time. Before I knew it, Casey was six years old and my watchfulness had shifted seamlessly from little boy to big boy—from park swings and blowing bubbles to organized sports.

Casey started playing soccer in the first grade; it was coed. The girls would stand on the field in groups of two or three, holding hands and plucking dandelions. When the ball came their way, they'd giggle. The boys would run after the ball in energetic packs, tripping over each other's ankles as they all vied for the same kick that might skip along in the direction of the appropriate goal. After fifteen or twenty minutes of this hodgepodge scrimmage, it was time for snacks. And there would be Casey, running full speed toward the bag that held the pretzel rods, in a faster sprint than any on the soccer field that day.

Scott and I laughed. *That's our boy!*

We were parents. How incredible. We'd never dreamed when we first got married that someday we'd sit on an elementary school field and watch our son run. Everything about Casey was a surprise and a delight.

As soon as Casey was old enough to understand sentences, we made it a point to cuddle up with him and recount his own special adoption story; I had put together a scrap book with drawings, photographs, and details of the day we flew to Texas to pick him up. Casey's adoption soon became a natural part of our family history. There was no reason to hide how it was that we had come to be his parents. But there was reason to hide something else from him—or to protect him from it as much as possible. The secret we kept from our son was the true story of what my transplant was doing to my body. Casey didn't have to know how sick I felt each day. There was no need to alert him when I went to the hospital for a heart biopsy or started another round of antibiotics to treat my latest infection. If I could keep smiling and do all the mommy things that Casey expected, why burden him with the truth? A three-year-old boy doesn't have to know his mother is not well; neither does a seven-year-old or a ten-year-old. All things in good time. The best mothers are the ones who know when to hold a thought.

"I bite my lip fifty times in the course of a day," a friend once told me, speaking of the new challenges that she faced as a mother of a teenager. "I literally bite down—front teeth into bottom lip. Otherwise I'm going to say too much, tell him something he doesn't need to hear. My son will survive even if I don't point out how unhappy I am when I see his jeans hanging halfway down his butt."

And Casey too would survive—and thrive—if I didn't share how my body felt each day. By age five, Casey knew from the scar that ran down my chest and from my cabinet full of medicines that his mother had undergone a heart transplant before he was born. But he also knew from my daily exercise and my seemingly endless energy that his mother was not fragile; she just went to the doctor a lot "for checkups and stuff."

"I'm fine, of course," I told him after returning from a late-night visit to the emergency room (a friend came to stay with Casey while we were gone). "Just another one of those silly mommy things. Had to check it out, just to be safe. Everything's great."

By the time his soccer games had become all-boy events with a ref in stripes and only a short half-time break for water, our efforts to protect Casey from the fallout of my heart transplant had become second nature. Scott and I hardly had to explain an ER visit or even a few days' stay at the hospital. As far as Casey was concerned, Mom was doing just fine—as always.

Only sometimes—not often—Mom would cry at the strangest moments. Once, she cried at a soccer game. She'd been sitting in a fold-up chair by the side of the field, watching the action intently and cheering just enough not to embarrass number eleven out there—her son. Dad was out on the field, helping signal changes in ball possession. Then one of the other boys got hit with the ball, right in the middle of the back. Hard. It knocked the wind out of him. The boy went down. The coach jogged over to him at an easy pace (if the coach had broken into a run, or if the boy's mother had dashed onto the field, it would only make things worse). Once down on his knees, the coach gave the boy a few tough-love pats on the back and helped him to a sitting position; the boy lifted his hand to signal that he was okay, he just needed a minute. Then the boy stood up, wiped his nose on his forearm, and strode back to his position on the field. The crowd applauded.

I cried.

I also clapped and smiled, emotion welling up in me for those who fight the good fight and force themselves up from the ground. But even as I brought my hands together for a boy I did not know, I was struck by a selfish thought: how nice it would be if someone could give *me* a round of applause from time to time when I rose from a fall—like after an encounter with the defibrillator paddles or in the middle of heart spasm on the angiogram table.

"Why are you crying, Mom?" It was halftime. Casey came to my chair to grab the water bottle I kept cool for him.

"It's just the sun, honey. Makes my eyes teary."

"You can wear my sunglasses if you want." I'd been holding them safe for him in my bag.

"Now there's an idea! Thanks."

My son was old enough now to wear sunglasses—kid-stylish ones with a cord that went around his neck. He was also mature enough to offer them to his mother, whose eyes looked like they needed some shade. But Casey would still believe a quick fib about the sun and proceed on his merry way.

He was a happy soccer-playing kid. Scott and I could take some credit for this; we were great parents.

Some tiny part of me was still left to wonder, despite myself, what would have happened if I had decided to get pregnant and carry a child. Would I have remained healthy through the pregnancy? Would the baby have done well even with all my medications? Answers could only be found in the stories of other heart-transplant women —some beyond the walls of Columbia—who'd gone on to give birth after their surgeries.

I heard through the hospital grapevine that Marissa went on to have a second baby post-transplant. The first child must have been all right and so opened the door for a second one. A few other babies had been born to heart-transplant women across the country as well, and I would read articles about them in magazines like *People* or *Redbook*. It was pretty much the same story each time: young woman, lifesaving heart transplant, healthy baby, healthy mom. At nearly sixteen years after my surgery, pregnancy was more of a possibility than ever for women like me because there was more data available to inform their choice. The media reports seemed so encouraging I thought maybe Scott and I should go ahead and take the pregnancy plunge, give Casey a sibling. But then I remembered the numbers—hard cold facts imparted to me by Dr. Davis when we first spoke about pregnancy— and realized that a handful of documented post-heart-transplant births, successful though they may have been, are not enough of a statistical sample to support a smart decision. Five post-transplant babies, ten, even fifteen, were not sufficient to drown out Dr. Davis's warning words about the "carrier" and the "fetus" as they played in my mind over the years. The crux of his message was: when it comes to a life, never take a bigger risk than you have to. And really, there would be two lives at stake if I were to get pregnant: mine, as the carrier whose carefully dosed medicines would be thrown off by hormonal and immunological changes during pregnancy, and my unborn child, as the fetus who —unfortunately—would partake in my daily immunosuppressives by way of the umbilical cord.

Scott and I had done the right thing by adopting Casey. We counted our blessings. And while I could not follow the progress of the babies born to the heart-transplant women I'd read about in magazines, I was able to track Marissa's well enough to see a longer term outcome. A few years after Casey's adoption, one of the transplant nurses told me that Marissa's elder child had developed a strange and serious illness. The fate of her second-born was as yet unknown. If this weren't enough of a fright to reconfirm our decision about the way we had become parents, there was an astounding phone call to hit the point home. It came out of nowhere one evening from Dr. Ganz; the soft-spoken arrhythmia specialist who'd cared for me in the hospital while I was on the transplant waiting list. Sixteen years after he'd ushered me to the transplant that would save my life, Dr. Ganz called to ask me a question relating to my sister, Jodie. She'd been having some arrhythmia problems and had recently become his patient. In order to provide treatment in the most comprehensive way, Dr. Ganz would need to tell Jodie some details of my medical history. New privacy laws in health care required him to obtain my explicit permission first.

"I need to be able to tell your sister about what they found on the autopsy of your heart," he said.

"Huh?"

"You do know that an autopsy was done, don't you?"

I did not. Sixteen years after my transplant, and I was hearing about it for the first time. "You do know what they found?" he asked.

I could only make an educated guess. "A virus in my heart? The Coxsakie virus?"

"Well, not exactly. I guess Dr. Davis didn't discuss it with you after your surgery."

"No."

"I'm surprised."

I wasn't. The last thing on my mind in the early days after my transplant was the fate of the diseased organ that had been taken out of me at long last. In line with Beverly's story about the flaccid liverlike heart that had been brought out to the waiting room in a metal pan, I'd imagined that the surgeon had carried the bloody thing back into the operating room after the show-and-tell and tossed it into the trash without a second thought. Now Dr. Ganz was setting me straight.

"Well, Amy, the autopsy showed that you had arrhythmogenic right ventric—oh, never mind the big long name, you had a congenital heart defect that was quite serious. Very extensive. It's something you must have been born with and lived with all your life. Eventually it caused your heart to fail."

"But I had a virus. They found a virus."

"There may have been a virus at work, yes. But your heart problems started when you were born, not when you contracted the virus."

I drew the phone away from my ear and stared down at it, mouth agape, eyes blinking wildly.

How could I have been sick all my life and not known it? I'd gone for check-ups with the same pediatrician every year when I was a kid. He listened to my heartbeat; he pressed a cold stethoscope against my chest and back. Why didn't he realize that something was wrong?

Because, Dr. Ganz explained in his gentle way, this kind of defect is almost impossible to discover; even an EKG won't pick it up. In most cases, the first time it is identified is during an autopsy.

"So a person has to die," I said.

"Yes. Often it will be a sudden death in a seemingly healthy person. Frequently a young person. An autopsy is done. The defect shows up. That's how this thing usually works; the diagnosis comes after the death. But not in your case. You got a new heart—and then they found the defect."

In other words, I had been saved even before the doctors knew exactly what they were saving me from. It's a rare patient who gets to have an autopsy performed on her heart without having to die first. The timing made me more than just fortunate; I was an anomaly. A different sequencing of events in my life could have produced a tragic result; an energetic sprint uphill at summer camp could easily have killed me when I was just a child, but it didn't. The severity of my defect had been of such grand proportion that my heart's ability to withstand it for so long was, as Dr. Ganz put it, "no small wonder."

A miracle?

Maybe even that. For the first time in sixteen post-transplant years, I could begin to see the journey of my heart illness in an entirely different way. Up until this conversation with Dr. Ganz, I had thought of myself as a woman who, at the tender age of twenty-four, had been the random victim of medical misfortune. Now it seemed that perhaps just the opposite was true: soon after my birth, I was singled out to be saved. Somehow I had lived into my early twenties without dying from a heart defect that could have taken my life much earlier. Not only had fate protected me from a premature sudden death, it also shielded me from years of psychological torment; since my body never gave me the sense that I was living with a dangerously malformed heart, I did not waste a single day of my youth in apprehension, waiting for this heart to fail me. These days of seeming wellness were a gift. They allowed me to amass an arsenal of sweet memories that would stand strong against the unsure times to follow. And when my heart finally became too sick to hide its insidious defect, it was not a tragedy in the way I had believed. It was just the arrival of an unavoidable illness that had been staved off by a long run of miraculous good luck.

It was as if my heart had put on a damn good show for me so I could enjoy a few more years of innocence. It also did me the favor of allowing medical science the time it would need to catch up with what would be necessary to save my life. If I had needed a heart transplant ten years earlier, I probably would have died; heart transplants had only just begun to be routinely successful right around the time when I needed one. With this good fortune in mind now, and viewing the onset of my illness through its new prism, I could no longer continue to see myself as having been *struck down*. For the first time ever, it seemed to me that I had in fact been *held up*—until it was the most opportune time for my body to fall. The fall itself had always been inevitable.

For the same reason, many of the mistakes that had been made by some of my doctors had also been inevitable—perhaps so much so that they should not really be called mistakes at all. Dr. Ganz hadn't made a medical error when he'd taken me off the anti-arrhythmia drugs for one night; nor had he been wrong when he'd put me on the electrophysiology testing table. He'd made these decisions based on the best diagnostic information available to him. No amount of careful thought or review of my case could have led Dr. Ganz to discover a dangerous heart defect that was undiscoverable. The best he could do with the knowledge he had was to assume that the devil behind my sick heart was a virus because that was what the tests had shown; there was no way for him to suspect that he was dealing with a genetically deformed heart until the surgeon held the culprit in his hand. My heart was sicker than even the most brilliant sleuth of a cardiologist could have known.

Dr. Bradley too had been deceived by my secretive heart. When he'd diagnosed me as having a heart virus "on the mend," he might have been correct. A virus that settles into an already damaged heart—one that has been struggling with a structural defect for twenty-three years—is never going to mend; it can only become part of a rapid deterioration and then be blamed for the ultimate heart failure. Dr. Bradley truly believed that the virus would play itself out and leave my heart to repair itself. But an episode of ventricular fibrillation had told him my illness was not progressing as he'd thought. When he called me at the hospital in Philadelphia and said, "You're a very sick girl, Amy," these words might have been as much a surprise to him as they were to me. And if this were so, it wouldn't have been his fault.

So doctors need to be forgiven. They cannot be omniscient. The treatment of disease is riddled with all kinds of unknowns. That my heart was able to hide its defect from two highly skilled cardiologists was not a fluke, it was a reality—one that I would now have to accept. There was no unpardonable oversight on the part of my doctors that had helped the destruction along. What happened to me demonstrated that there are illnesses that can outsmart and outperform even the best doctor gods in New York City. This would be a difficult truth for me to swallow, since I was still a patient very much in need of the kind of doctor who exists only in wishful thinking: the doctor who knows everything and is always right.

"I appreciate your telling me this, Dr. Ganz," I said, feeling more shocked than grateful, "though I have to say I wish I'd known about it sooner."

"I understand, and I'm sorry about that. But you know, if a reason came up where you needed to have this kind of information, I'm sure Dr. Davis would have given it to you. Like if you decided to get pregnant. You'd need to see a genetic counselor."

Ah, the effect on the fetus. Yes! It was not just the cyclosporine that stood between me and a risk-free pregnancy after all. There were genes involved. If I had decided to go against Dr. Davis's advice and become a "carrier," he would have been forced to reveal the genetic issues. But why hadn't he simply opted to tell me earlier? If he had shared all the facts at the outset, it would have shortened our pregnancy talk by years. Perhaps Dr. Davis had thought it more important to set my sights ahead—on law school and its successes—than back into the past.

"Now that your sister is my patient, I'd like to tell her about it too," Dr. Ganz said. He and I both knew that Jodie and her husband had decided against having children. Still, he wanted her to know that, as my sister, she too might have a defective heart; although in her case, the malformation must be significantly milder than mine had been. Jodie was in her forties and her heart was still quite healthy, except for some arrhythmia that responded well to medication. In all likelihood, she'd already gotten safely through the testing period that would have ratted out a very sick heart. Still, Dr. Ganz wanted to keep an eye on her, just to be safe.

My sister was going to be okay. But the wheels of my mind had already begun to spin away from Jodie, turning my thoughts closer to home—to how this new information affected me and my life. Its implications began to take shape. If I had in fact gotten pregnant, I might have been the one to carry on the bad seed that had been planted somewhere back in my family tree. How unbearable it would be to give birth to a child who would go on to experience the anguish I'd been through. Even if this child were to be spared the genetic defect, he might then pass it along unknowingly to a child or grandchild of his own. This whole cycle of illness could have been propagated by the fulfillment of a wish on my part to carry a child, come what may.

I told Dr.Ganz that he was free to tell Jodie everything.

Thank goodness I hadn't gotten pregnant. Thank goodness Dr. Davis had held off my decision long enough for me to realize it was motherhood I was after, not the use of my uterus for gestation.

And thank goodness for Casey, my healthy boy who would never make me feel worried when he ran up a hill or across a soccer field as fast as he could.

24

AFTER HANGING UP WITH DR. GANZ, MY FIRST CALL WAS TO SCOTT. I reached him at the office and summed up what I'd just heard. He told me it really sounded fascinating, but he was very busy at work. Could we talk more about it in an hour or so when he got home? I said that would be fine and moved swiftly to my next call, Beverly, who always had lots of time for me.

I took her through the conversation step by step.

"You had a virus," she said, even after I'd finished explaining what Dr. Ganz had just told me about the small role that the virus had played in my heart's ultimate failure.

"I had a birth defect."

"A virus?"

"No, I'm telling you now that it was a defect. I was born with it."

"No one said anything about that. Only about a virus."

"That was before the autopsy."

"What autopsy?" I'd just told her all about it.

"The one that showed a genetic defect."

"But you had a virus in your heart."

This conversation was going nowhere. Beverly refused to allow any change to the diagnostic story she'd settled on years ago. For some reason, an errant virus was a more palatable culprit—in Beverly's view—than an insidious defect. I asked her to put Dad on the phone.

I relayed the new information again, hoping for a clearer reception.

"What defect? There is no heart defect in our family," my father said. "Except maybe your grandmother—on your mother's side." My grandmother had developed artery disease in her old age. But my heart's abnormality had nothing to do with occluded arteries.

Apparently, my father wasn't hearing me either. I had expected that he and Beverly would share in my amazement on learning these new facts so many years after the original diagnosis. The true origin of my heart's demise was a stunning revelation. I was bubbling over with newfound perspective and longed to share it with someone beyond Scott. I wanted my parents to join in my surprise and all its effects. I wanted to go deep and wide.

They didn't want to go at all.

So I called Jill.

"You've got to be kidding me," she said, at once understanding everything I'd just told her about the autopsy news. "Oh, my God, this is major. It's got to change your thinking, right? I mean, wow!"

Yes, right. Wow. Jill got it—again. She was a courageous friend, eager to hear me with open ears no matter how unpleasant the subject matter. Jill listened better than my parents did—and without cringing.

"Thanks so much, Jill," I said.

"For what?"

"For saying the right thing. For listening so well."

I had other dear friends who would listen too, and just as intently. Later that night, I called each one of them in rapid succession, just to share. But I was aware that only Jill, the woman who gave me a teddy bear for my first hospitalization, and who had also been the little girl who sat beside me in my second-grade class picture, would understand enough to give voice to my feelings in just three perfect sentences: this is major . . . change your thinking . . . wow. Jill hadn't just listened to me; she'd heard me as well.

Something struck me just then—a revelation in the making, fragments of it coming together to form a thought I'd never had before: *Besides my family, Jill is the only person who knows what I was like before I got sick.* Scott and I had met only a few months before the cardiomyopathy hit; we'd barely moved into the toothbrush-sharing stage of our relationship when I was hospitalized for heart tests. The Amy he would come to love deeply was not the same Amy that Jill had grown up with. Scott hadn't had enough time to memorize the contours of my true unburdened self and my smiling face before my illness, but Jill had witnessed them for many years: the second-grade photo, the fourth, the sixth, the junior high musical, the high school basketball game. Holding on to these images, Jill still remembered the healthy Amy she once knew. All my other friends—and even my husband—would never know what they had missed.

When Scott and I moved our lives and Casey's from the city to the suburbs, Jill and her family followed. So did three other couples who had been our closest friends. We all made it our business to settle in the same small town, hoping that similarly close relationships would develop and continue among our children as well. And just to be sure that the adult bonds stayed strong and special, we carved out time to spend together as a cohesive bunch—without the kids—on vacations that were absolute musts. We used fortieth birthday celebrations as the no-excuse hook to lure all five couples to the same spot at the same time. The celebrations, on average, popped up about once a year, and when they did, no less than eleven adorable children would be left at home with grandparents or nannies so that the lucky moms and dads could go away as one joyful, fun-loving cluster.

And what a fit, agile bunch we were, celebrating our way through vacation spots and scenic locales, some near, some far, but always an adventure of sorts, each trip tailored to the particular travel passion of the birthday guy or gal. We were, as a group, five globe-trotting, gym-loving, multiple-mile-running, healthy, successful men in their early forties, along with fitting counterparts to match: well-toned, beautiful-faced, elite-grad-school-degreed, spry, sure-footed women. But the husband-wife pairing was imperfect, thrown off only by one—the obvious birthday group clunker—and I was it: the sick girl, the one who didn't quite fit the pretty picture.

My friend Lauren was gorgeous as we set out for her fortieth birthday trip. She glowed with happiness as our group gathered at the airport, hugs and kisses circulating among us all. We were on our way to Spain for a week of birthday fun.

I was in for a challenge. Lauren's husband had given us an itinerary of the trip before we left, and I knew I was in trouble. At sixteen years post-transplant, I was going to find it nearly impossible to drag my body through the fast paces and intense summer heat of a multi-city jaunt through Spain. I knew from past birthday trip experiences that I would be the one—the only one—for whom this vacation would be more hard work than simple pleasure, because it required me to be something that I was not: healthy, carefree, and fabulously forty-ish like everyone else. While my friends could simply be themselves, I would have to rise up and push myself unmercifully, almost masochistically, to be much more than I could possibly be, just to keep up and enjoy.

Just to smile at the dinner table.

The itinerary daunted me. I went down the list with Scott and indicated the many activities and excursions where I thought I might fall short.

He wanted to solve these problems for me before they arose. "You don't have to go to the running of the bulls." (Or to the late-night suppers where the appetizer course would not reach the table until 11 P.M., or to the long hours walking the heat-scorched sidewalks of Barcelona in search of art or a carafe of icy sangria I would not be allowed to sip along with my thirsty friends.) "You can just tell everyone you'd rather take it easy and stay back at the hotel. There's nothing wrong with that."

Except that I would be the lone member of the hypermobile group who would consider taking it easy. For me to act on Scott's suggestion would require that I, the sick girl, stand conspicuously and painfully alone.

Or, of course, I could ignore everything my body and my husband told me and forge on as if I were a full-fledged member of this select group of active, perfectly healthy people.

This was what I chose to do.

I bore Scott's I told you so's and joined the others for all the excursions, the most difficult of which was the trip to Pamplona to see the running of the bulls.

We all got up at four-thirty in the morning for a long drive that would get us into the city before the gates closed for the big event. In the pre-sunrise dampness, our group tumbled into a van, sleep-deprived, intent only on sprawling across a couple of seats and falling back into the scant hours of sleep we'd left behind in our hotel beds. All eyes were just half open except mine; I was busy calculating, staying alive. In about two hours, when we were due to arrive in Pamplona, it would be time for my morning medicine. This meant that when the birthday group dragged their exhausted selves out of the van and wished out loud, "Oh, what I wouldn't do for a double espresso!" I would have to hang back and swallow my medicine, shake my head a few times from the bitterness, and make a wish of my own (albeit silently) that I didn't have to live in a world full of people who didn't have heart transplants.

On arrival in the city, our guide told us to grab hands and run together in a flexible snaking line, one after the other. Soon we would be a birthday-group chain cutting our way through the unmoving crowd of cackling tourists and native Spaniards bursting with anticipatory vigor. We were dressed in white, all of us, from head to toe, with a splash of red in the bandannas we'd tied around foreheads or necks as we pleased; this was the required attire for anyone entering the city of Pamplona that day. And so our handsome chain of whites and reds began to wind its way along the cobblestone streets, under wooden barricades, over piles of garbage and vomit still left over from a week's worth of rambunctious merriment preceding the event, and through the chaotic maze of bodies and tightly spaced buildings that stood between us and our prearranged balcony. It was barely 7:30 A.M.

The cyclosporine was just beginning to hit. I needed to stop and rest, but I was a connecting piece, a vital link in an unstoppable, unbreakable procession. Our guide kept calling out for us to go faster, and then I would feel a tug on my arm, followed by an instinctive quickening of my feet into an all-out run. I was sure I was going to throw up whatever there was in my nearly empty stomach. Or pass out. I looked up at the chain link next to me; it was Jane, her smiling face held up to the morning sun. She was laughing, the bottom of her chin grazing the red bandanna looped fashionably around her neck and coming together in a smart, tidy knot just beneath her right ear. In front of Jane there was Rob, also beaming, shouting out some semi-Spanish words to urge us all on, in good, raucous, early morning fun: "¡Arriva! ¡Vamos! ¡El toreador!" And then there were Lauren, Lenny, Jill, Michael, and the others up at the front, leading the way, leaping forward with graceful, syncopated ease, like gazelles through the woodlands.

I was near collapse.

Turning my head to look back behind me, I searched for Scott, my unfailing source of energy; and there he was, looking very much a part of the birthday bunch, so handsome and European chic in his white pants and loose linen shirt. He smiled at me in a way that said, *Isn't this just the greatest?* and gave my fingers an excited squeeze.

No, this wasn't the greatest, not at all. Not for me; only for the sturdy sequence of people with whom I was linked, literally and inexorably.

The chain. The chain with one weak link, one nauseated, breathless, struggling woman who'd forgotten to put on her red bandanna that morning (but who'd sure as hell remembered to take her medicine). Nine gleaming pictures of health and one heart-transplant patient, and she could only be spotted—or ratted out—by an eye well trained to pick up on the most desperate of disguises. She was the one wiping tears aside with the back of her hand, super quick, before they'd fall and be seen. She was the one who was just as tired, if not more so than the others, but who'd said *no, thanks* to coffee on the balcony (only because she had to; even a small cup of coffee would surely make her denervated heart beat scary fast and wild). She was the one in the group photographs whose smile had a hint of grinding molars behind it.

After the bulls had finished their run, our group set out for a day-long tour of Pamplona. By 2 P.M., I was nearly broken by exhaustion. There was no amount of will that would overcome it, I knew, so I stifled my pride and gave in to the fatigue—even though no one else in the group seemed ready to call it a day. The reality of my heart transplant was about to rear its ugly inscrutable head, front and center for all my friends to see, and I would have the opportunity to watch their reaction to it.

"I have to go back to the van. Now. Right now." I tried to pull our tour leader, Pablo, aside so the whole birthday group wouldn't have to hear the urgency in my voice.

Since Pablo had been told in advance that there was a group member with a "health problem," he could swing into action quickly without asking questions; in a flash, he efficiently split off the healthy fold from the one person who would pull them down. Lifting his hands up beside his left ear, he clapped them together twice, tango-style, and made an announcement: "Hello, everyone!

Yes, hello! Amy, here, she needs to go back to the bus so she can rest." My friends looked up from their shopping bags, mildly bewildered but not particularly concerned. "I'm going to set Amy and Scott on their way, and I'll be back to all of you in a moment. We can go hunting for some more T-shirts when I return, if you like."

Scott walked along with me to the van and made sure that the driver was there to let me in and turn on the air-conditioning. Once I was settled on the long stretch of seats in the back row, he planted a quick kiss on my forehead and left to rejoin the others, but only after asking several times—with tenderness and care—if his departure was truly all right with me. I couldn't bring myself even to consider saying no to Scott; I'd slowed him down enough on this trip already, even before Pamplona; it seemed selfish to allow myself what I needed from him at that moment. Or perhaps it was more that I'd been silenced by the heartbreaking sense that even my loving husband's presence beside me couldn't make things all right today. I closed my eyes as Scott started down the steps of the bus. Only then did the tears fall fast and cool against my steaming cheeks.

When I awoke half an hour later, there in front of my just-opened eyes was Jill—the birthday group member who also happened to be my best friend since second grade. She stood at the end of the center aisle of the bus, waiting patiently for my attention, then plucked a T-shirt from a plastic bag and held it up to me by its shoulder points.

"I bought it for Casey," she said. "Thought you might want me to. I hope this size is good."

It looked about right.

"Candy?" She offered me my pick from one of the overstuffed treat bags that had been scattered around the bus for all of us to share.

"No, thanks."

"You okay?"

"No."

I could say this to Jill.

I knew she expected me to go on and say more, and so I did. "You know how it is, Jill. I feel like crap and I follow along all day like I'm fine. It kills me. I'm not like the rest of you guys. I have to try so damn hard. Too hard."

It was tears that cut me off just then, not a signal from Jill to rein in my honesty. There was no such signal. Nothing about her wide, encouraging brown eyes and tender smile told me she'd heard enough.

"You should know that you did really great out there today," she said. "It was tough even for me. I could barely stand up half the time. And I'm not taking medicine that makes me feel sick all day long. I have no idea how you got yourself up for this crazy day to begin with. You are amazing. Truly."

"Yeah, so amazing I had to come back to the van."

"Believe me, I would have loved to come back with you. I was all too ready to lie down about an hour ago. Really." Jill had in fact offered, earnestly, to take Scott's place and accompany me to the van, but I'd refused. "Okay, I know you have a heart transplant and everything, but don't think for a minute that this is an easy trip for any of us. We're all exhausted. And oh, my God, for you to do what you've done today—hold up the way you did, and for so long—you have nothing to be ashamed of. Besides, you missed absolutely zero. The T-shirt stores made for pretty shitty shopping. Not worth it at all."

Even if this weren't true, it was still nice to hear. I brought my eyes up to meet hers in a moment of best-friend connection that had no limits on candor.

"But at least you had the strength to go shopping," I said, hitting her between the eyes with my heart transplant.

Jill didn't draw back at all. Instead, she leaned in for a hug, "Oh, Amy. You don't have it easy, do you?"

"No, I really don't."

And then we sat for a long time, my friend and I, after the others boarded, holding hands in silence as the van made its way out of Pamplona and through the winding scenic hills of the Spanish countryside.

25

ONE SUMMER LATER, IT WAS TIME FOR ANNUAL EXAM NUMBER SEVENTEEN. Dr. Waller was there beside me again—just as in all the years before—as I lay on the narrow table, covered in sterile sheeting. Scott sat in the waiting room as usual. Cath lab nurses with familiar faces moved around the room busily, some of them taking a moment to call out a compliment intended to put me at ease: *You always look so terrific! Wish I had your figure! Oh, that beautiful hair of yours!*

Only Mary—the nurse who'd been there with me for more exams than any other—knew I was too anxious to take in any well-meaning flattery. She stepped toward me and leaned down for a private moment. "You're shaking," she mouthed silently.

"You know I always do."

"Are you cold?"

"No. I just hate this."

Mary reached under the sheet and gave my hand a firm squeeze. She smiled up at Dr. Waller and nodded once, signaling the okay. My exam would begin now.

Dr. Waller turned immediately to his usual tricks, engaging me in light but irresistible conversation while threading a catheter through a small incision in my neck. This was the early part of the biopsy, where I was still allowed to speak, which meant that I could be lulled merely by responding again and again to the voice of my tried and true cath lab doctor seeking me out, if only to talk nonsense. But just a few minutes later, I would have to turn completely silent and still. In most years, we would see each other only once, Dr. Waller and I, for about an hour, on the day of this annual exam, which meant there would be a lot of catching up for us to do within a short span of time—in between catheter snips at my heart and measured releases of dye into my bloodstream. And at the end of our get-together, we would both come to know in an X-ray instant whether or not my heart had taken a turn for the worse in the last twelve months.

Dr. Waller continued to pepper me with rapid-fire questions. Just after wiping the side of my neck with some antiseptic, he prattled on intently, moving through the seasons of the year gone by and touching on each of them in swift succession that would barely allow me a few seconds of silence to focus on the way his hands fussed above me.

He asked if I'd traveled anywhere special over the summer.

"Ouch!" Dr. Waller had timed this question perfectly with the first needle stick.

"Sorry." He jabbed me a second time and then a third, real quick, just to get the anesthetic injections over with. "Sorry, again. And again."

I took in a deep breath and exhaled the stinging pain. Dutiful patient that I was, I redirected my attention immediately to the question Dr. Waller had just asked me, ever willing to feign unawareness. He was my favorite cath lab doctor, after all; the one with the most conversational tongue, sharpest wit, and most dexterous hands. The least I could do was play along with his earnest efforts to move beyond his own white coat and keep the nonmedical gab going for the sake of my cath lab comfort.

"I went to Spain last July, with the fortieth birthday group. You know about them."

"Yes. The lucky bunch. Ah, summer in Spain. Did you run with the bulls?"

"Well, as a matter of fact, I—."

"Quiet. No moving now. Pressures." It was time to take the first measurements of the pressures in my heart. After many years of annual exams, I still did not know what this meant exactly, but I understood it was a clear signal for me to be still. I allowed my mind to drift off as the nurse called out the numbers (pressure measurements) and documented them either on paper or directly onto a computer, I could not tell which. I was lost under the sterile plastic sheet, eyes closed, thinking back on the summer trip Dr. Waller had just brought up in my memory. I let my mind wander so that time on the exam table might pass more quickly.

Yes, I'd been to the running of the bulls. . . .

"And did anyone get, you know, gored? Trampled? Any of that sort of entertainment?" Twenty minutes had already gone by. Dr. Waller was now finished with the biopsy and back to his incessant questioning. Today it had taken him only eleven separate delves into my neck (I counted)—only eleven plucks at my heart muscle—before he'd come out with the four pieces he needed. It was a good day on the biopsy table.

"I saw a couple of people get head-butted," I said. "You know, with the horns?"

"That must have been fun."

I felt the tap on my thigh: angiogram time. Dr. Waller always moved seamlessly from one invasive test to the other as if both were part of the same procedure, but they weren't. Whereas the biopsy was done through a vein in my neck, the angiogram centered around an incision in an artery in my groin, and the thigh tap meant that the first shot of dye was now on its way into my bloodstream. I felt it run its customary path up to my forehead and back down as usual, but today it stopped—or, rather, lingered for a few moments, somewhat pleasantly—in my crotch. Out of all the angiograms I'd had over the years, only a scant few had ended in this dye-induced delight, a rush of intense unnatural warmth. Sometimes it happened, sometimes it didn't. But when this feeling graced me with its fleeting presence,

I'd call out *Woo-hoo!* and Dr. Waller would know just what I was crowing about. Then there'd be some witty back-and-forth about "holes" in the groins, "little pricks," (referring to the small needle injections he'd made before inserting the groin catheter), and the hidden pleasures of coronary angiography.

Today was one of those *woo-hoo* times. I laughed myself to silliness, a captive audience whose mind had given way to the potent combination of Benedryl (to promote a comfortable drowsiness) and Valium (a narcotic kicker) that I'd opted to take before the angiogram. But then the first picture of my arteries came up on the screen, and the cath lab turned silent.

"What do you see, Dr. Waller?" It was not an easy question to ask.

Without enough hesitation to render an informed opinion, he tossed back an answer, clucking. "I see your arteries, Mrs. Silverstein. What else would I be looking at?"

This kind of levity could mean anything, coming from him. In this moment, it meant that Dr. Waller was stalling for time as he tried to figure something out. Good news couldn't take this long, I thought. Even through the effects of sedatives, my whole body began to tremble in sync with the staccato of molars clacking in the back of my skull. Then I slipped into my compulsive habit of running numbers while on an exam table. I wanted to believe that this kind of thinking would ease my anxieties, but somehow it always turned into instant fodder for the hunger of my worry mill: *Let's see now, I'm seventeen years post-transplant; that's sixteen years after my wedding; seven years past my life expectancy. . . .*

I was not calmed.

"It's gone." Dr. Waller's voice muffled my thundering mind like a heavy blanket. "Wow," he said simply, and then again, "Wow," without any of the emotion or excitement one might expect to come along with two distinct *wows* in a row.

"Wow what?" I couldn't help but shout.

"The changes on the right side—the ones that have been there for years—I don't see them today. Of course, I have to take a comparative look at the films, but it looks like they're gone. Wow." His voice remained flat, unnervingly listless.

And yet he'd just given me the very best news I could hope for: a seemingly spontaneous reversal—or disappearance, even —of artery disease (the "changes" he'd just cited) at seventeen years post-transplant. For a reason I could not yet begin to fathom, my most reliably chummy, chatty doctor appeared to be pulling back from my shining moment of post-angiogram glory. In a flash, Dr. Waller, my cath lab pal, retreated into the kind of rote disconnection I had come to expect from all the other white coats in my life.

He turned on his heel, stony faced, with the tight crisp pivot of a soldier. As I still was not allowed to move from the table, I rested my cheek against the pillow and watched the side view of Dr. Waller striding to the other side of the room, where he began to remove the X-ray protective garb from his chest. In previous years, this post-exam lull had been prime time for jokes and giggly banter. But today there was an awkward, cavernous silence. I longed to break it—to bring the final moments of this annual exam into line with the ones that had preceded it in years past.

"Hey!" I called out, as he headed toward the exit door. "Thanks —and I know you know what I mean! Thanks for ripping out pieces of my heart and sticking a plug in my groin and filling me up with premium octane kidney-killer dye."

I expected a laugh. Or a Waller touché. Instead, I got formality. Distance.

"Anytime, and you're quite welcome. It's always a pleasure, Mrs. Silverstein."

What?

In the final moments of annual exam number seventeen, every last bit of fun had been sucked out of the cath lab by a piece of *unexplainable* good news.

Why?

Because of the discomfort that springs from medical situations filled with a mix of unfathomables. As pleased as Dr. Waller must have been with the disappearance of vasculopathy (the first signs of which had begun showing up on my angiograms years earlier, but had not progressed beyond a safe level), he was also unnerved by it. The patient whom he counted among his favorites, and whom he'd known for the longest time, was now proving to him in a bold way that the fate of her transplanted heart, good or bad, was beyond the comfortable range of medical predictability. Maybe even beyond the scope of his knowledge entirely. This could only mean that it was best to get out of the firing zone of the cath lab before I began shooting off questions he would not be able to answer—or, worse, didn't want to answer, like "Does this test result mean I can stop worrying about transplant artery disease?" and "Am I finally safe?"

Dr. Waller would have to tell me no, I wasn't safe, but that he did not know exactly why this had to be, it just was; heart recipients always wound up with irremediable artery disease (transplant vasculopathy); that's just the way things went for patients out there like me. But Dr. Waller knew as well as I did that there weren't many—if any—patients quite like me. There were gaps in the statistics as well as in the science of heart transplantation, big ones, and I was the kind of patient who always seemed to fall right through them and down into the black hole of the unknown. This was why Dr. Waller scurried away from me today—and why I had to let him go.

I'd decided long before my seventeenth annual exam that I would never fall into the trap of thinking of doctors as friends. My relationship with Dr. Waller may have teetered on the edge of camaraderie, but I would always catch myself before reaching the point where I believed that having his beeper number meant there was an actual friendship between us. We were silly, witty pals, that's all. Anything more than this was bound to lead to disappointment.

Because I knew firsthand that when illness begins to spin out of control, doctors will show themselves to be just that: doctors, capable of achieving tremendous self-serving distance in record time.

I first learned this lesson from my beloved internist, Dr. Clark. Severe cardiac illness swept my body up and away from him, and he had let go. He must have known when he sent me for urgent testing on that Friday night that I would not return again either as pal or patient; when a young woman becomes seriously ill, she must leave her comfy internist forever and enter the bleak world of the specialist.

As a general rule (and a surprising one to people who would have no reason to know any differently—or any better), internists are, in essence, doctors for healthy people. In my healthy pre-transplant early twenties, I assumed—quite naïvely—that my huggy doctor would be mine forever. I had pictured many years of jaunty checkups in Dr. Clark's office and found safety in believing that, if something bad were to happen to me, he would be by my side to the end. But as soon as the reality of my cardiomyopathy diagnosis hit, I was swiftly delivered from his familiar care to the impersonal poker-faced management of the cardiac specialist, Dr. Bradley. What I'd assumed would be just an adjunct to my core relationship with Dr. Clark would fast become the whole of my medical care. I fell into the forced change unaware at first and then resignedly, once I realized that a permanent handoff had been made. Dr. Clark must have wanted it that way, I thought, and took it more personally than was warranted. It did not occur to me at the time that I had become too sick for the care of a generalist, even the "best" generalist in New York.

But I learned fast. Soon after my surgery, I became a quick study on the logistics and procedure of doctor hopping and the crawl up the specialist ladder. As I continued to make this climb year after year, I reached a point where I could look back and view Dr. Clark's unannounced secession from my medical care as a first lesson in the importance of maintaining the dividing line between doctor and patient. I realized in retrospect that there had been only a continuous dialogue between me and Dr. Clark during those cozy office visits: never a friendship. The camaraderie was a self-serving illusion that could not survive the somber diagnosis of cardiomyopathy.

If I hadn't felt so devastated by the departure of my beloved internist, I might have recognized the great and prophetic favor he had done for me by demonstrating what not to do when forming relationships with doctors. Because of him, I would never allow myself the illusory comfort of another Dr. Clark, no matter how cuddly-warm, no matter how inviting. As a heart-transplant patient, I had no choice but to form ongoing relationships with more than a dozen different doctors, but I was careful not to become too fond of any of them. Occasionally, when a doctor acted in a way that felt a little too "Dr. Clark" for my liking, I would pull back abruptly. Like the first time Dr. Davis returned a phone call and identified himself using his first name.

I picked up the phone and heard his voice on the other end, prosaic as ever. "Hello, it's Ron. How are you feeling?"

"Oh, hello, *Dr. Davis*. Thanks for getting back to me." There was no way I was going the Ron route with this guy.

But my emphatic rejection of Dr. Davis's effort to be on a first-name basis had no effect on him. Year after year, phone call after phone call, he would tell me (in so many words), *You can call me Ron*, even though time and again I insisted, *No, I can't.*

Ron could not be the name I would use to address the man who might have to tell me someday that I was dying and there was nothing he could do to save me. If and when the time came when I would have to be told such news, better to hear it from Dr. Davis than Ronnie baby. My interactions with Dr. Davis could never be informal because I could never for a moment forget that seeming calm in my transplant body one day could easily become wild illness the next. The way I saw it, vigilance had to take the place of friendship on all levels, even in the names we used to address each other.

A few years after my transplant, Dr. Davis returned a call I'd placed with his answering service on a Saturday afternoon and then I wound up at Columbia's ER late that same night with a cough, nausea, and a high fever. Early the next morning, he came by to see me, standing at the foot of my bed and looking on, close-mouthed and expressionless. I might have expected more empathy, a showing of emotion, or some tender words, like "Oh, you poor, poor dear!" But what I wanted even more was a smart, quick mind that could figure out my medical problem and make it better; this man at my bedside was my transplant doctor, after all, not my nursemaid.

"What's wrong with me?" I asked him, my head down, hair falling forward as I continued to choke and cough over a clean plastic bowl that had just been placed in front of me.

Dr. Davis answered, in a voice as empty as his eyes, "I don't know."

I lifted my face up and looked at him in disbelief.

He shrugged. "I'm not a lung specialist." There was a spot on the wall behind my head that seemed to be a magnet for his eyes. Gazing right past me, he continued on in a blank tone, "You have a cough. Dr. Schultz needs to see you. I'll call him."

I craned my neck forward and gave him a hard stare that was part entreaty, part bafflement. I'd become well used to the idea of specialists by this point, but it was the first time I had ever encountered unabashed, openly admitted ignorance on the part of the sure-footed Dr. Davis.

"You don't know?" I asked, woozy with nausea.

"No. Okay? Bye," he said, matching three short words with three long strides as he slipped out the door. His giraffe legs carried him high above the unmanageable, daunting jungle of my hospital room and delivered him safely into the hallway—where his white coat would have some meaning again.

There goes my lifeline, I thought, and threw up.

A difficult truth came to light on this day and would show itself with regularity for years to come; Dr. Davis did not feel sufficiently competent to treat my lungs (or sinuses, or kidneys, or skin, or any other aspect of my body that suffered the effects of transplant immunosuppression) because he was not a specialist in these fields. Fair enough, but then I would expect that the specialist he recommended would take over with confidence and get to the bottom of my problem. This, however, would not be the case; a quick glance at my list of medicines was all it took to spook some of the most self-assured and high-credentialed specialists in New York City. These were doctors who were supposed to know it all but who knew only enough about heart transplants to recognize that I presented a challenge beyond their comfort level. Whenever I'd receive a diagnosis from one of these bigwigs, it would always come hand in hand with a panicky disclaimer that cut them down at their Ivy League legs—and they resented me for it.

"I can only guess here. You're immunosuppressed—on cyclosporine, for crying out loud. With a patient like you, it's hard to be sure about anything." This was the usual cry. In other words, if this superb specialist was not able to help me (or even if he wound up harming me a little), it was not a reflection on his talent and reputation as a celebrated physician. Instead, it was my fault.

The more well-established the specialist, it seemed, the greater the effort to self-protect. I'd witnessed some of the most esteemed doctors in New York throw their hands up—literally—and resort to a cowardly ego-saving maneuver I came to call "the punt." This tactic was evident whenever I'd present a doctor god with a problem that fit squarely into his specialty but was, of course, intertwined with a puzzling transplant element, such as a high likelihood of infection.

The doctor would barely hold the challenge in his mind for a single minute before tossing it back to Dr. Davis—the very doctor who'd told me "I don't know" in the first place.

"What does your transplant doctor think about all this?" The punt.

"He told me to ask you."

"But he's the transplant expert."

"But you're the specialist. Dr. Davis is a cardiologist; he deals with my transplanted heart. And my heart is fine. I'm here to see you for a different part of my body."

"But you're immunosuppressed. Don't you have a doctor for that?" Attempted punt.

"No."

"Well, I'll make my best guess here. But I gotta say, you're a wild card." Fumble.

The ball drops at my feet.

Dr. Davis had started the toss in the first place, and then the specialists threw the quandary back again, complaining that there were things they shouldn't be expected to know. I was left in the middle. There was well-educated guesswork, there was conjecture based on the highest medical intellect, there was even out-of-the-box round-table-type theorizing on the part of truly well-intentioned doctors, but never was there an *answer* to any of my post-transplant medical problems. The illnesses that managed to get resolved did so in spite of never having been diagnosed and understood in the first place; and the ones that never really went away—but only faded into the background and then reappeared with regularity—were chalked up to the unavoidable dark side of transplant life. Even the ways in which I managed to stay healthy for seventeen years remained unexplained mysteries that challenged my doctors and made them feel uncomfortably less than omniscient.

Like the apparent disappearance of my artery disease—a piece of good news. With a quick telephone call, Dr. Waller punted to

Dr. Davis, whom he expected to come speak with me in the recovery area.

Within minutes, I heard the familiar stride of long legs in loafers across the tile floor. The curtain opened and there was Dr. Davis, smiling a rare smile. In all the years I'd looked at the features on this face, I'd never seen teeth before.

"The changes on the right appear to be gone. Great. I am pleased," he said, in dry measured blocks of sound that proved for the first time that Dr. Davis in fact could inject true gladness into the smile on his face, if not into the timbre of his words.

I couldn't resist pushing him a little. "What made the changes go away?"

He shrugged his shoulders playfully, wide grin still firmly in place.

But I was not kidding around. "No, really, what did it?"

"Good clean living . . . I guess."

"But I've always lived good and clean, you know that. I haven't been doing anything different. How can I stop my arteries from getting diseased again if I don't know what I did to get rid of the disease in the first place?"

Dr. Davis lost his smile. His lips became two horizontal lines.

"I think we should switch you over to a new medicine," he said. Apparently, medical research had led to some refinements during the seventeen years since my surgery, and now there were alternative immunosuppressives preferable to my current regimen. One of the most vital drugs I had been taking all this time, Imuran, had become a near anachronism. Dr. Davis wanted me to start taking the new equivalent instead, CellCept, a medicine that had proven more effective in suppressing the immune system and staving off transplant artery disease.

"But why would I switch now, when I'm doing so well?"

"Because we want to *keep* you well."

"What are you saying? Do you think my arteries are going to clog up all of a sudden?"

"I don't know."

There it was again: uncertainty, damn it. And, worse, this time Dr. Davis was being tentative about how best to protect my transplanted heart, the very organ about which he was supposed to have all the answers.

"Well, if you don't know then I'm not switching," I said. "How do you know the CellCept will work better for me? How do you know it won't wind up wrecking my arteries or giving me some kind of transplant cancer?" Cancer—especially lymphoma—was a side effect of this type of immunosuppressive drug, both the Imuran I'd been taking and Dr. Davis's recommended replacement.

"I guess I *don't* know."

The furrows in Dr. Davis's brow grew noticeably deeper. He paused, brooding over my words as if close to doubting his own wisdom in having suggested the change in the first place. For me, there was not nearly enough certainty in Dr. Davis's reasoning to support a medicine switch; maybe there wasn't even enough of it for him.

Dr. Davis stepped away from my stretcher, shoulders slumped, hands sliding deep into the pockets of his white coat. "Look, I'm telling you this because I've only got a few heart transplant patients who've made it as long as you have, and they've developed serious artery disease. I want to do everything I can to make sure you stay healthy."

"But I thought my arteries were really good. You said they looked great, right?"

Time to punt. By now, Dr. Davis had backed all the way up against the curtain at the entryway to my cubicle. "See you later, when they take you upstairs to your room," he said. His body was out of view now; only his head poked its way through the opening for the final word. "And, yes, your arteries are okay. We need to keep them that way."

The bedside talk that had begun in the recovery area concluded several days later in Dr. Davis's private office, where he told me that his suggestion to switch medicines had been "just an idea" and the final decision would be mine to make. Never before had he placed something so important in my lap. Not sure what I was supposed to make of this transfer of power at first, I soon recognized Dr. Davis's statement for what it really was: a punt—the first one he'd ever sent in my direction. I accepted it as an honor. Dr. Davis was not trying to bow out of his role as my decision-making doctor; rather, after seventeen years of dictating my medical regime, he was now asking me to engage with him in a discussion—an exchange of thoughts on a question that, admittedly, neither one of us could answer with total confidence.

So we talked. There was a calm but sharply pointed back-and-forth: I told Dr. Davis that I would not allow the demonstrated success of the new drug as used in *recently* transplanted patients to suggest that there would be similar results in patients who'd survived for seventeen years—at least not without proof; he countered with a rejection of my rationale for sticking with my current medication—If it ain't broke, don't fix it—but then admitted to me that there had in fact been no studies on the effectiveness of the new drug in long-term heart-transplant patients. This admission on his part led to some softening on mine; I opened my mind to the idea that there had been some real advances in transplant medicines over the last seventeen years and it might be possible for me to benefit from them.

We conferred until it became apparent to both of us that there was no "right" path to take. There was no one way to save my arteries—or my life.

I had to make a choice. But when I finally decided, I didn't feel that I had made this choice alone. In the end it had been based on the combined best efforts of two intelligent minds, mine and Dr. Davis's. Or maybe even mine and Ron's.

I decided to stick with the old medicine.

26

Two months after my annual exam, I came down with a sinus infection, this one only days after I'd finished a long course of antibiotics for the very same illness.

My sinuses became badly infected almost monthly due to the perilous combination of immunosuppression and my natural-born occluded nasal passages, and each time I'd have to take a string of transplant-size doses of antibiotics (at least twenty-one days) in order to fight it off.

My first sinus specialist was a young cocky star player for the Columbia head-and-neck surgery team. He told me that surgery was not merely an option for me, it was an absolute necessity and I could die—*die*—if I didn't let him—and only him—operate immediately. He seemed gleefully intent on scaring the hell out of me, insisting that sinus infections in transplant patients were likely to spread rapidly to the eye or brain; I could wind up with meningitis or some other wild infection that would run amok and take my sight or my cognitive function before even the most powerful antibiotic could make an inroad. Then he reached into his trove of horrors and pulled out a little story about my transplant friend, Ellen. "You probably remember her, right? The one who died? I saw her the night she came into the emergency room. Knew right away it was too late for that girl. Infection in her trachea. Jeez. It could've started with a sinus infection. Who knows in a transplant patient? I had to cut her throat open, *trach* her, right? Man, what a shame. If only she'd paid attention to her symptoms earlier, I could have saved her. Ah, well. You know how it is, I'm sure."

He looked at me with one eyebrow lifted in that spooky Vincent Price kind of way. I shuddered. This doctor seemed all too pleased, his wry smile giving away how much he was enjoying the effect his ghost story had on me. Smugly victorious in what he'd set out to do, he hurried me along to the reception area and barked at his secretary, "Book her for later this week, first day available—emergency endoscopic sinus surgery."

"This week?" This was all happening much too fast. I hadn't even talked to Scott.

"You don't want to end up like Ellen, do you?"

No. But I wasn't going to trust the word of this self-promoting fearmonger doctor without a second opinion, and maybe even a third. That's how I came to meet Dr. Allen, a conservative physician, measured and calming in his approach. He too was a sinus specialist, and a head-and-neck surgeon as well; he could have rushed to operate but didn't, saying, "Let's give antibiotics a fighting chance, shall we, before diving into a nasty surgery?"

The next fifteen years would be filled with antibiotic fight—but to no avail. The infections were coming faster over time and more virulent than any drug could manage, and I wound up back where I'd begun years earlier: facing the imperative of sinus surgery. Finally Dr. Allen operated, hoping that, if all went well, the infections would stop. It didn't happen, though; soon after surgery, I came down with a sinus infection just like before. And then, it seemed, another one, not long after my annual exam.

Again, I wound up in Dr. Allen's office. But this visit would not be routine.

Dr. Allen told me to remove my "blouse," please. It took me a few seconds to understand that he was referring to my turtleneck sweater, and then I quickly drew it up over my head and dropped it into my lap just as I realized that I wasn't wearing a bra; I'd been at home, in pajamas, all day. Dr. Allen hadn't offered me a hospital gown because there wasn't one in the room; sinus examinations didn't routinely involve the removal of any clothing. But this was an emergency visit. If in the next few minutes my doctor was able to feel with his hands what I had felt deep in my armpit with mine—a round, hard mass—it could mean cancer.

Naked from the waist up, I sat high in an elevated dentist-type chair, with my breasts falling just below the eye level of a doctor who ordinarily would have no reason to see them. Dr. Allen pressed two fingers far up into my armpit, then opened his eyes wide as saucers and gazed up at the ceiling. He appeared panicked even before his fingers reached the palpable lymph node—the axilla—and when he finally landed upon it, his eyes closed tight as if something had just caused him great pain. He winced.

"Yeah, yeah, I feel it," he said, withdrawing his fingers and bringing them together with the rest of his hand to wave away my nakedness. "Put your blouse back on."

Here it was: post-transplant lymphoma. Cancer.

I couldn't find my breath. Fumbling with the edges of my turtleneck, I finally managed to locate the hole at the top and poke my head through. Dr. Allen didn't wait for me to pull the rest of it over my chest before he began barking out a string of urgent directives.

"Get dressed. Get on the phone. Call your transplant cardiologist. You need to biopsy this lump—now. And I want you to have your bone marrow tested at the same time. You don't want to waste one minute, believe me."

Another emergency. I'd been through them before. But this one felt different, and within seconds I realized why: this time I was alone. I had gone to see Dr. Allen on my own today; there was no one out there for me in the waiting room. Scott was at work, unconcerned, because that's the way I had been as well; neither one of us thought for a minute that today's doctor visit would end in cancer hysteria. I'd simply done what I'd been doing since my transplant: indulging in self-examination; my throat was terribly sore, so I pressed against the sides of my neck to see if my glands were swollen. Then I'd checked under my arms as well—a reasonable thing to do in the case of flulike symptoms and sore throat—and found something there. I wasn't sure what it was, but I knew I should run it by a doctor. Since Dr. Davis was away on Christmas vacation, I'd chosen a familiar specialist on my own, and the closest thing I could find to a cancer doctor was my own sinus specialist, who performed surgery on necks frequently as well. I'd grown to trust Dr. Allen's honesty, if nothing else. Today, I had expected that he would examine me thoroughly as usual, say that there was nothing serious going on under my arm, and send me on my way. But instead he launched me into new and dreaded territory: oncology. First, though, my transplant cardiologist would have to be notified.

I told Dr. Allen that Dr. Davis was out of town. "It's Christmas week. No one's around at Columbia except for my transplant nurse, Sara."

"Get her on the phone, then," he said, opening the door to the examination room and disappearing quickly into the hallway. Soon I could hear animated talk coming from the next room; Dr. Allen was telling his assistant about me. The word *lymphoma* was used more than once—emphatically.

I knew I was supposed to get up and make my way to the telephone on the wall, call my nurse, and explain the situation to her so that Dr. Allen could then get on the line and give further instructions—but I was frozen in place. I couldn't bring myself to begin the process of fighting cancer, not even the diagnostic phase. To start down this road would mean breaking a secret promise I'd made to myself soon after my transplant: *I will fight through the little illnesses, and I'll even do the bigger ones if I have to, but never again will I fight the enormous diseases—the killers that are going to get me no matter what I do. I won't take on another one.*

Lymphoma was something I was not willing to take on. Still, the question remained. Would I put myself through the steps that would determine whether the lump under my arm was in fact cancer? Diagnosis would require surgery. Apparently this kind of lymph node could not be biopsied in section, the entire node would have to be removed. For a transplant patient like me, this would involve a risk of infection. It could also mean carrying two illness-based identities at once—heart-transplant patient and cancer patient—at least for a while. Perhaps to my death.

Dr. Allen slid back into the exam room on his heels. "Did you call your nurse?"

I stared down at the floor, ashamed of what I would have to tell him. "I can't. I mean, I won't. I can't do cancer, Dr. Allen."

"Oh, sure you can. You had a heart transplant. You're strong."

"No."

"But you're such a brave soldier! You can do this, easy. Don't be ridiculous. I'll telephone your nurse myself if you like." He called out to his assistant to get Sara on the phone right away.

"No. I'm not a brave soldier. I don't want to be a soldier at all. I've fought my battle for a long time. It's been grueling . . . and tough . . . and unwinnable. I'm exhausted. I've done the heart transplant thing so damn well I'm still alive seventeen years later, and I guess that's my victory. But I am not just an infinite heap of courage. I'm a woman, Dr. Allen, a thinking, feeling woman. I have my limits like anyone else—and I think I've reached them."

I was asking a lot from Dr. Allen. I was asking him to accept something that no one in my life ever could: I was indeed a brave soldier, but there was some suffering I simply would not abide. There was a point at which I would choose not to take bodily abuse anymore. This was incomprehensible to others. If a woman were indeed strong enough to withstand a heart transplant, extensive infections and arrhythmias, horrible exams and hospitalizations, and all the rest of the things that would make the average person recoil, why wouldn't she choose to fight cancer too?

No one doubted that I had the ability to forge on, so they all expected me to do so, almost automatically, because, simply, *if you can, then you do.*

I could, but I wouldn't. And to people in my life—friends, family, and doctors—this made me seem irrational, even crazy.

Dr. Allen wouldn't hear of it. "You don't know what your limits are, Amy. People fight. They do it all the time."

"You don't know me, Dr. Allen."

"I don't know *you*?" he said, chuckling to himself as he dropped down onto a low stool in the corner of the room. "You don't know *me*." His elbows slid forward on his knees and he leaned toward me, hands clasped tight together. "I would like to tell you my story, if that would be all right."

I was not sure it was, but something soft in his eyes made me nod.

"A few years ago I found a lump in my neck. I showed it to my partner down the hall, a throat guy. He thought it was just an abscess, but I knew it was cancer. I had it removed, and I tell you now it was a bad, rare form of cancer, the worst kind, that kills you fast. A five-percent survival rate. I shut down my practice and called the kids home from college. Their father was supposed to die, right? But as you now see"—Dr. Allen brought his arms out to his sides while lowering his head in a sort of humble bow—"here I am."

But the road had been unexpectedly long. He'd lost nearly sixty pounds along the way. His liver failed. He was admitted to the hospital several times in the wake of each chemotherapy treatment, only to be treated with disrespect by the same doctors with whom he had once walked the hall as equals. "I hollered at one of these guys—a resident who didn't know what he was doing—and the next thing I know there was a psychiatrist at my bedside! Everyone thought I was some kind of agitated nut. But I wasn't crazy; I was enraged because I couldn't believe I was ever going to get better with some imbecile for a doctor. And you know what I did? I put my clothes on and got out of there—left the hospital and took a cab home. My wife couldn't believe it when I walked in. She was so upset with me."

Scott too would have gone mad if I'd done something like that. He would make me go back to the hospital and apologize in person to every doctor, nurse, or aide who'd even gotten a whiff of my anger, regardless of whether I'd had to put up with a total fool of a resident assigned to my case. Scott might even side with the dim-witted psychiatrist. But here was Dr. Allen, another brave soldier like me, apparently, only he'd become battle-weary and had gone AWOL long before he'd accumulated seventeen years of fighting under his belt.

"But you know, Amy, I never gave up. This is the thing—and I say it to you here and now." He reached down and took both my hands in his. "As long as you live you must fight. Always fight."

"But I've already fought."

"It's not something that begins and ends. You must see it as a journey. Life is a journey, Amy, hasn't anyone ever told you that?"

Yes, I'd heard the journey thing before, sure, but never from a doctor. No one in a white coat had ever bothered with something that had no science to it, no numbers, no diagnosis. Talk of journeys was the stuff of that darn pesky "discomfort" that always made doctors either scurry away from me or punt like mad. But Dr. Allen stuck this one out, partly because of what he'd been through himself, but also because of the person he was. The man. The soul. Dr. Allen was not my friend, but he had a friend's staying power.

He kept his other patients waiting and held my hands tight until he could tell that it was okay to let go. Then he got my transplant nurse on the phone and instructed her on the exact details of the next few steps of my care.

Soon I was out the door with a knowing wink from my doctor and a written list of everything I needed in order to move forward.

"Good luck," he said, handing me a slip of paper.

And I was off on my next journey.

27

ANYONE CLOSE SHOULD HAVE KNOWN THAT MANY YEARS OF BUILT-up emotion was about to explode inside me. But no one did. Even Scott failed to understand fully how the accumulation of health problems had worn away my resilience and devoured my sense of hope. Transplant illnesses are not discrete events that come and go in tidy succession. They were my everyday life. The suspicious lump under my arm did not happen in a vacuum; it occurred within weeks of my coming smack up against two other complications that were equally menacing—recurring infections and an annual exam that forced me to choose between my doctor's advice and my own instincts about a vital medication. Now, as I awaited a surgery that would tell me whether or not I had cancer, I felt myself suffocating. There were too many things wrong with me, too many illnesses and health issues vying for my urgent attention all at once. If I could have put one of them aside for a while—just one—maybe I wouldn't have felt so desperate to escape my own body. But heart-transplant patients don't deal with just one medical disaster at a time. I was destined to be overwhelmed—and bound to fall.

And so I fell—down, down—into the dark place where people go just before they give up completely. In the three days between my office visit with Dr. Allen and the scheduled surgery to remove my lymph node, I allowed myself to take a good, long, contemplative look at the body I would be leaving. This required me to abandon my seventeen-year effort to keep myself distracted from how sick I felt every day. Now I would do just the opposite; I would pay close attention to how awful it was to be me. There would be no need to fight my way through the debilitating side effects of medicines anymore. Instead, I would do the unthinkable and the uncharacteristic: lie down on the couch, close my eyes, and allow myself to feel my transplant body in all its insidiousness. I'd abandon the usual mind-set that had allowed me to carve out rainbow arcs of fabricated optimism. I would not try to find comfort in Beverly or Jill the way I always had before when illness crushed my spirit beyond recognition.

Then there was Scott. If I was going to spend the days leading up to my surgery reducing my existence down to a hell that encompassed only a wretched body and my feelings about living in it, I would have to put Scott's love aside. Closing my eyes to his radiant light was the only way I could experience total darkness, and this was a most unnatural thing for me to do. I would have to act quickly now before he lifted me up again. I told Scott flat out to keep in mind that I had agreed only to have the lymph node *removed;* if the biopsy showed lymphoma, I would kill myself immediately; he could be sure of it. With this statement came a blackness that eclipsed everything bright and inspiring about Scott that had pulled me through in the past. And this darkness propelled my determination to break down and spiral inward. Now was the time to shed illusions so I could know for once what my body and mind felt like when I did not cling to empty optimism through self-distraction. Only in this way could I decide whether I truly wanted to live or die.

I shut my eyes and concentrated on the latest sinus infection that was now laying siege to my body.

The exhaustion was not the kind of tiredness that the average person might feel when hit with an illness, crossing time zones on a whirlwind business trip, or running fifteen miles without proper conditioning or training. Mine was a sick-girl kind of exhaustion, the result of a combination of immunosuppression, infection, and nauseating medicines. It made for a degree of depletion that could force a person to collapse into complete inertia. I'd had this feeling hit me many times before, though I would always try to put it aside: while driving my car on the highway; in the middle of lunch with a friend; halfway through building a sand castle with Casey on the beach. Always it was a signal that an illness was on the way; I was about to get very, very sick. I would tell Scott later on how hard it had been for me to finish what I was doing when the telltale fatigue hit. The onset of infection made me feel like my body was being sucked into the ground and I'd had to use every ounce of my willpower to overcome it—as if I were a normal person who felt a bit ill and had to wait a while before taking to bed. Once or twice, Scott, the unfaltering and remarkably uncomplaining recipient of my "I didn't feel well today" stories, said to me, "You couldn't possibly feel that bad. It's like you're the only person who has ever felt sick. You always make it sound like it's the worst illness that there ever was in the world. Look, I get it—you don't feel well. There's no need to exaggerate just to make the point. It's bad enough that you're sick again."

This would prompt me to make a feeble attempt to explain to him, perhaps in a different way this time, what it feels like to be sick and immunosuppressed. I had played the role of the perfect heart-transplant patient for so long that even my husband seemed to have forgotten what my body was up against. He needed another gentle reminder, and I knew I would have to keep my emotions in check as I slid this one by him. "I'm sorry to correct you on this, honey, but I have to. Please hear me out," I said, proud of myself for not screaming *You don't understand!* and storming off in a fit of anger. "I know it seems like I'm making a big deal of this, but I'm not. Honestly, it's much worse than I let on. It's a kind of sick you can't possibly know, because you're normal. I used to be normal once. I remember what sick felt like without a heart transplant. It was nothing like this."

Another failed attempt at explaining myself. I allowed my words to trail off, culminating in a nearly inaudible *never mind* under my breath. When Scott let his eyes glaze over the way he did then, I felt he didn't understand me, didn't believe me. Or maybe the truth was something worse: maybe Scott was just plain tired of hearing his sick wife drone on, month after month, infection after infection. Even the most adoring, compassionate, kindhearted man needs a break after so many years of steady round-the-clock listening and bottomless empathy. Scott was tired too.

Maybe it would be good if I just died already, I thought. As I lay in bed contemplating what might be revealed by the upcoming lymph node biopsy, I began to consider the possibility that a diagnosis of killer cancer might be the best thing for everyone involved. It seemed somehow unnatural that I should still be alive so long after transplant. Everyone was weary, and my medical problems had become a big yawn to those who looked on. A ten-hour emergency-room visit—complete with medical errors and finally, a hospital admission, at 3 A.M.—no longer piqued interest or elicited sympathy. It was just something Amy did. *There had been seventeen years of it, for heaven's sake.* A surgery no longer warranted a phone call from a friend. *Why bother? Amy does them all the time.* Lymphoma? *Well, these things happen.*

It had gotten to the point where even Scott had taken to rolling his eyes at my complaints, not because of their drama but rather from their relentlessness. His was more a look to the heavens than a call for calm rationality, and I knew this even as I saw his eyes lift up and flutter. Scott felt terrible (not just for himself but also for me) that having a heart transplant meant I could never feel well for more than a few hours at a time; but man, was he tired of it. This began to show around the corners of his eyes. If I had died five or ten years after my transplant, as I was supposed to, Scott and the other important people in my life would not have gotten to the point of losing all patience. An earlier departure would have been a more graceful exit, like when a football player, afraid of losing his fan base, bows out of his career before his game begins to deteriorate. But I was seventeen years into my career as a heart-transplant patient, and it seemed that everyone had watched me long enough to lose interest. The grand game of life went on, but I didn't figure in it much anymore.

This was how I saw it from the new vantage point of my living room couch, the big ugly secret for those who have no idea what it is like to be young and permanently sick. Everyone else's life goes on. There are fun parties and great trips that go ahead without you. There are others you are able to attend, but you're so sick when you do, it's almost as if you weren't there at all. You look at photos of yourself at these events and remember how hard it was for you to put your face up to the camera and smile. But no one knew, because you wore your mask, the one that turns you into a perfect heart-transplant patient who refuses to drag a good party down.

So while the people around you continue to get a little drunk on the latest chic cocktail, you sip sparkling water, hoping it might make you feel a bit better, but it never does. Then ten o'clock rolls around—time to take your immunosuppressives—and you know that once you swallow them, you'll feel a hundred times worse: guaranteed. The idea crosses your mind—oh, it sure does—that maybe you'll just skip your medicine tonight. But no, you're a good transplant patient, a compliant sick girl. You don't fuck with instructions. That's one of the reasons why you're alive today—here at this fabulous party, this trip, this restaurant—with all these healthy people who would fall to their knees and puke their guts up if they had to swallow the venom you're about to place in your mouth—again.

Gulp.

Down it goes. You've just made it possible to live another day, so you can wake in the morning and repeat your poison.

Was I the only heart-transplant patient to think of my lifesaving medicine as poison? From the moment I introduced my body to a whopping dose of immunosuppressives, I could feel it recoil from what the chemicals were trying to do. I sensed at once that something was dying inside me, grabbing at my throat, lungs, and abdomen until I could swear I heard my insides crying out *What are you doing to me? Stop!* as the dose of toxins began to kill off my beautiful immune system. What had once been an integral and vibrant presence in my body—all those lovely white cells and T cells, cancer fighters, common cold repellants, and virus sentries—was now the enemy of the pills I'd just tossed into my mouth. Every day without fail, twice a day, for seventeen years I'd felt this war coursing through me and was sickened, not just by the physical side effects but also by the disturbing thought that I had to poison the most health-giving system in my body in order to stay alive. It seemed that when I agreed to a heart transplant, I had made a deal with the devil; in return for one precariously healthy, pulsing organ, I would endure a lifetime of poison and all its ill effects.

As I faced the possibility of a lymphoma diagnosis, I felt ready to see how far I could push my end of the bargain. The idea of trying this out was not new—it had occurred to me before—but now the specter of cancer had given me a prime opportunity to put it into action. As far as I was concerned, if the biopsy revealed cancer, all deals were off: the deal with the devil, the deal with Dr. Davis, and the deal with the perfect transplant patient within me—the one who wanted to be a wonderful wife, a steadfast mother, and a well-masked sick girl. This deal had included my promise to take my medicine every day exactly as directed and without question. The amount of medicine (and therefore the level of immunosuppression) was at the sole discretion of Dr. Davis, chief antirejection wizard and administer of poisons. I had asked him many times in the past to please, *please* lower my medicine levels, but he'd refused. I told him I couldn't stand the infections anymore and I really needed to feel well every now and then, but he wouldn't give in. When I pointed out that I hadn't had a single episode of rejection in all my years since transplant, and it seemed counterintuitive that my body would reject a donor heart that had been part of it for so long, Dr. Davis got all steamed up and adamant: I was on the lowest possible dose of medicine, he said, and there was nothing more to discuss.

But the discussion had continued in my own mind for many years and I decided that, when the time was right, I would lower my medicines all by myself—maybe even to the point of stopping them completely—and see what happened. It took a somber diagnosis like the possibility of lymphoma to set this medicine-lowering plan into action. In the winter of 2005, I readied myself to test my fate.

It had been quite a journey that brought me to this point of desperation. I arrived at rock bottom with a loud thud, letting everyone know that Amy was down and this time would not be making her usual impressive attempt to rise above her illness. She was just going to lie on her couch for a day or two—and stop trying.

It was a very *un*-Amy thing to do. I knew it was selfish and ungrateful—after all, I was lucky just to be alive. Any lapse in the way I embraced my good fortune as a transplant patient was viewed as unseemly by the people who'd come to expect better from me.

No one liked me much without my sugarcoating. My popularity was assured only so long as I played the role of ever-resilient patient. My friends had realized long ago that when Amy started "talking nutty," going on about how she simply must cut her medicine levels down—and without her doctor's okay, no less—it was time to end the phone call, leave the coffee shop, ignore her morbid musings entirely, and start an upbeat conversation about the new shoe store in town. I found I had full control over the comings and goings of the people in my life based on how resistant I was to the temptation to remove my mask and be honest about living with a heart transplant. It was okay if I said I didn't feel well—and I could even cry a little. But any talk about messing with my medications was sure to repel even my closest friends; it sounded too much like suicide. Once I went over to the dark side of my transplant self, I would find I was suddenly alone. Whether I opened myself up or lied my way closed, loneliness was always waiting for me at the end.

Scott hated it when I said I felt alone. How inconsiderate of me. My feelings of loneliness made him think his presence didn't make much difference. If I could still feel isolated when he was right there by my side, I must not be appreciating his presence. And hadn't he been there through it all? Every emergency-room visit, every annual exam, illness upon illness, doctor after doctor? Almost all the memories of terrible medical moments since the onset of my cardiomyopathy included the strong, clear presence of Scott—holding my hand, stretched out alongside me on a hospital bed, calling a doctor in the middle of the night, wrapping his arms around my shaking, feverish body until I was all cried out. I would surely have shriveled up and died without him. He'd been as close to me as he could possibly be, and yet I still felt lonely—because, in my heart-transplant body, I *was* alone.

Even the greatest love is powerless to overcome the connection between serious illness and loneliness. Built into the doctor visits, hospital stays, and diagnostic tests are pockets of isolation. When Scott drove me home from a medical procedure, the details of the experience were already pretty much over for him. But for me they would live on. I remembered how the needle hurt, even though the doctor said it wouldn't, and how I'd been promised a hand to hold during the really hard part of the exam, but for some reason the hand never found its way to mine. Memories of a doctor saying, "Oh, no, not good!" halfway through a procedure, and then ignoring me when I asked him what he meant—this was the kind of alone that never went away, not even in Scott's loving presence.

And now I had to go into surgery without a word from the doctor I relied on and trusted the most. Dr. Davis was off in California.

I could not understand why Sara would not find a way of contacting him for me. She finally admitted that there were strict rules against bothering cardiologists when they were on vacation. The only chance these doctors had to really get away was to allow them to relinquish all responsibility for their patients—even the sickest among them—during these precious holidays.

But it's *me!* I wanted to say to Sara. "Dr. Davis wouldn't mind having his trip interrupted for *me!*

As if she'd heard what just passed through my mind, Sara added, "He doesn't take calls from anyone when he's away."

But I wasn't just anyone. I was Dr. Davis's perfect transplant patient. I did everything right. I'd never failed him. Wasn't I his favorite? Hadn't I earned it? Didn't he love me just the littlest bit after all this time? It couldn't possibly be that Dr. Davis would want his most treasured patient to have surgery without his input. There was no way he would want me to face the threat of cancer alone, right? Couldn't Sara just call him for me—tell him Amy needed to speak with him, that there was a possibility of lymphoma?

"I suppose I could e-mail him," Sara said, "but I don't know if he'll answer."

This was encouraging. It seemed to me that Dr. Davis was the kind of person who would check his e-mail even during vacation. Surely he would call me when he read about what was going on. If I could just hear his calm, sober voice I'd feel better. Sometimes just having him recite in dull flatness what he wanted me to do was enough to give me the strength to do it. I felt less alone when following a definite path set for me by Dr. Davis. As long as he and I were together in my struggle against illness, I could rise up and be the best heart-transplant patient ever.

Sara received a return e-mail from Dr. Davis the next day. He said I should see an oncologist. That was all.

A punt.

28

After three days of lying on the couch, I got up. I had to. A stronger part of me responded, finally, to the call of obligation—most of all to myself. I realized that the light I'd shone on my own body with decisive intensity over the last few days had failed to reveal anything I didn't already know. My transplant life was hard. Very hard. But I had survived many years of it—sometimes scrambling, and other times coming as close as a sick girl could to soaring. With this endurance came a sense of pride. I was not about to quit now, to let go of the rope of my life before I knew whether post-transplant lymphoma had finally made it impossible for me to hold on.

I pulled myself together for the surgery.

Once inside the pre-op area, I was my usual brave transplant self with my perfect-patient mask fully in place. Scott sat on a chair beside my stretcher and looked on, curling his lower lip under his front teeth while two nurses prepped me. I told the nurse where to find my best vein and reassured her, lightheartedly, that I was famous for "easy access." It was a far cry from the first time an IV nurse had come my way at New York Hospital seventeen years earlier; dozens upon dozens of IV insertions later, I'd learned from repeated experience that the best way to get a needle into my vein on the first try was to set my own jitters aside and put the nurse at ease. Today I would be rewarded with the ultimate compliment. "You're a terrific patient, you are! A pleasure!" she said, in a singsong voice, and slid the needle into a plump compliant vein just above my wrist bone—painless, like a dream.

Soon it was time for Scott to leave the pre-op area. He kissed me quickly on the lips, as he'd done on all the other occasions when I was about to be wheeled away, and then slipped out the door unceremoniously. I'd gotten into the habit of becoming smugly courageous, to the point of near indifference, at the moment when Scott left my side. There was no amount of affection sufficient to offset what was in store for me, so why bother trying to dredge anything useful out of my last few seconds with him? Better simply to remember his face (which I'd always found to be glaringly beautiful at times like this), shore up my strength, and accept once again that I was alone.

I anticipated that there would be a brand-new gruesome medical memory created today and I would have no choice but to add it to the others without being able to share its details with Scott—or anyone—in a meaningful, visual, sensory way. I'd wasted my breath too many times trying to relay my impressions of illness and death to people who, ultimately, would disappoint me by proving that they'd been hardwired only for processing information that supported their ignorance and showcased the brighter side of modern medicine. How quickly my friends and family could turn my threatened lymphoma into the equivalent of their own medical experiences: a cough that hung on for more than a week, cosmetic surgery, a sprained wrist, a stiff neck. These were the kinds of ailments that most often had happy endings that made the tough parts worth it—like having to wait for the results of a pregnancy test after trying to conceive a baby for three whole months. The people closest to me, whose understanding would have been invaluable, could only run my ordeals through their own filters and then invent wildly far-fetched, impossibly upbeat conclusions that had no basis in my reality as a heart-transplant patient. Their creativity had more sting to it than they would ever realize, but I knew they called it up for a good cause: optimistic nonsense about my health situation made everyone feel so much better. Except for me.

This was why most times it was easier for me to be alone. By myself in the pre-op cubicle now, I sat upright on the stretcher and pulled my knees in toward my chest. It was a sort of self-hug I'd taught myself years before, during the many long weeks spent waiting in the hospital for a new heart. Visitors would come and go all day, every day, but there had been many hours when I was left alone with only a book I was too sick to read, a television set I was too weak to watch for very long, and the ominously erratic beats of my heart monitor for company. If I listened to my heart sounds for too long, I began to imagine them coming together to form a death march. Terrified that I might die without having someone there beside me whom I loved, I came up with a way to create a second presence that would be with me in case my heart petered out before or after visiting hours. I discovered that, thanks to my small torso, I could reach my arms all the way around, back past my narrow shoulders, and place my hands against either side of my spine to create an embrace that would always be available to me. Positioned this way, I would pat myself on the back with wide open palms that made hollow thumping sounds, calming me as they echoed through my rib cage. Then I'd speak aloud in a voice that was more breath than sound: *There, there, Amy. You have such a hard road. Too much for one girl in one short lifetime. No one should have to do this. . . .*

I found myself wrapped in this kind of solitary hug today, with nearly the same words coming from my lips. But this time my self-hug had the opposite effect; its loneliness and desperation led me into an all-out deluge of tears. Just as I disintegrated into an all-out weep, one of the nurses threw aside the curtain at the far end of my cubicle and caught me, mask off, arms enveloping as much of my body as they could. I let go of this pose at once, falling back onto the stretcher.

"Oh, dear, you're crying. Look at that, the top of your gown is wet with tears. Here, now, take this." She handed me a small pack of generic hospital tissues—the cheap, scratchy ones I hated—and placed her hand on my forearm. "Why the tears, honey?"

Did she have to ask? Come on! I was about to be wheeled into a surgery that would reveal whether or not I had cancer. "It's nothing, really. I'm okay. Just feeling a little sorry for myself," I said.

"Of course you are, dear. With a heart transplant . . . and now this surgery today. Well, you just let it all out now, why don't you." A second nurse showed up, the one I'd spoken to when I first arrived. She appeared confused by the sudden change in my demeanor. Her colleague set her straight: "Amy is feeling sorry for herself, wouldn't you know. It's okay for her to feel that way, don't you think, Helen?"

"Sure. Oh, yes. It's a lot to deal with. A lot for her—for you, I mean, Amy." She touched my cheek lightly with the back of her hand. "I'd cry too if I . . . you know . . . had to do all this." Her eyes shifted to the bag of saline hanging on the IV pole beside me.

Their sympathy was all I needed to dry my tears and turn self-pity into resentment faster than I could blow my nose. I was protecting my honor—my precarious place among normal folk in society.

Soon it was time for me to go into the operating room. I swung my legs off the side of the stretcher and stood up; I was going to walk into this surgery on my own two feet. The nurses protested and told me cheerfully that I should just "go for the ride!"

"Only sick people ride," I said.

One tug at the back of my hospital gown to pull it closed behind me, and I was headed down the hallway, sliding my IV pole along the floor, propelled by the very last bit of my pride and determination. An empty stretcher followed in my wake.

* * *

The surgeon called me a few days later with preliminary results: the excised node was benign. I didn't have lymphoma after all. A tremendous weight had been lifted, which left me feeling more willing than ever to carry the daily burdens of my heart transplant—at least I didn't have to carry cancer as well. It was as if I'd been tapped on the shoulder and reminded that things could be worse. Now I knew they weren't, and the sense of relief was profound.

But I was still in a lot of post-surgical pain. I was not expected to feel this badly one week after the operation, but there had been complications: things that were not supposed to happen in the wake of the removal of a single lymph node from my underarm. Perhaps I was the person least surprised by the unlikely problems that ensued from this simple procedure. I'd learned years ago that my transplant medicines could make all sorts of bad things happen—even when they weren't supposed to.

A single small needle-draining of my armpit one week after surgery should not lead to a hematoma—a painful swelling of blood forced from the vessels and diffused beneath the skin—but in my case it did. Just an hour after leaving my surgeon's office, I rushed back in again as an emergency patient with an agonizing, bulging mass of blood that needed immediate opening. The still-raw scar under my arm would have to be cut open so that the insides could drain, and then the wound would be reclosed. It was a second surgery of sorts—in a doctor's office rather than an operating room, because of the urgency. And I wasn't put to sleep this time; the agony was fully palpable. I wailed my way through the waiting room and onto the examining table.

My poor surgeon hadn't appreciated what she was up against from the start. "I take out lymph nodes all the time," she said, "and in thirty years this has never happened to me." She appeared to be genuinely dumbfounded, if not a little embarrassed—clearly distraught for her doctor self and sorry for me, her traumatized patient, at the same time.

I looked down at the cupful of blood-tinged yellow fluid she'd just drained from my armpit. "Nothing happened to you. It happened to me," I said, squinting at her through laughing eyes to show I was just playing around with words. I wasn't really upset about what had happened, was I? I'd be a fool to alienate the surgeon whom I would have to visit once or twice a day for the next week so she could drain the heck out of my armpit with a needle as long as a butter knife. And besides, I had no reason to be angry with her; she'd performed the operation perfectly, and with the genuine kindness and empathy rarely seen in a surgeon of her high status and reputation. It was not this doctor who had failed me; it was, once again, my complicated, immunosuppressed body that let me down by turning something routine into a great big deal.

My underarm was still a fiery mess of needle holes and a twice-stitched incision when the day arrived for my appointment with Dr. Davis. Scott was going to accompany me to this one, but first he had to go to work. The original plan had been for Scott to drive his car up to Columbia straight from the office and I would meet him there at the end of the day, but neither of us considered that I would have to navigate south on my own with one hand on the steering wheel; even a hairline shift of my left shoulder still felt as if the skin beneath my arm would rip open straight through to the bone. But Scott and I had made a plan and I would stick to it, no matter how painful. I let my bad arm lie motionless in my lap and crept along the highway at half speed, turning a simple thirty-five minute trip into a long, difficult hour.

I arrived before Scott anyway. He called me on my cell phone to say he was stuck in traffic and would be late; could I ask Dr. Davis to wait for him before getting to the more important parts of today's discussion? But I knew there would be no way to begin this conversation gradually; once I had Dr. Davis's full attention, I would be like a racehorse out of the starting gate. I'd been waiting for this opportunity since Dr. Davis had crushed the last bit of my spirit with his careless vacation-time missive, showing me in one cold sentence that to him I was not worth a five-minute phone call. In the week that followed his pivotal e-mail, I had spent three pre-surgery days in my stupor and then underwent a lymph node excision that led to a complication under my arm and nearly a dozen painful fluid-draining sessions with a surgeon who'd never seen anything quite like it. And now, as I was about to come face-to-face with Dr. Davis for the first time since he'd hung me out to dry, I felt about ready to burst. To hell with small talk and delay tactics while Scott sat in traffic on the West Side Highway.

Sorry, Scotty.

A shadow fell over the magazine that lay open on my lap. I looked up and saw a silent Dr. Davis towering over me, the top of his head blocking out the light and nearly grazing the waiting room ceiling. He was, as always, running right on time for his appointments, even though I was the last one scheduled for today. Most doctors would have been way behind by now, but not him; he always moved patients in and out of his office with deliberate speed.

I, however, was never intimidated by Dr. Davis's apparent disinterest in hearing me out; rather, I took it as a challenge and refused to let even his worst grimace deter me. It was my sense (or imagining) that Dr. Davis welcomed my tenacity and, perhaps reluctantly, respected me for it. My interactions with him often felt like a game or a test of will. It might have appeared that he wanted me to give in or give up and allow myself to be frightened away like the rest of his patients; but in fact Dr. Davis seemed just as pleased to have me stand my ground and prevail over his brusqueness.

I glanced down at my watch and calculated that, given Scott's location when he'd called me from his car, I was going to have about twenty minutes alone with Dr. Davis before he arrived. This would give me just enough time to hit my doctor squarely between the eyes before anything could stop me. I had assured Scott that he didn't need to come today (which would leave me more free to throw punches), but he'd insisted. It was one of those rare times when he felt worried enough to call my doctor on his own—even before I did—and set up an appointment for the three of us to meet. He'd tipped off Dr. Davis about the recent change in my attitude and outlook since the whole lymph node escapade had knocked me to the ground: I was feeling its reverberations and was talking "in extremes." Before Scott could fill in the details, Dr. Davis headed him off in typical fashion. "Bring her in on Tuesday. We'll talk," he said.

So I was to be brought in like a criminal into a police interrogation room? Oh, I was a lawbreaker, all right, and dangerous, with my angry, smart mouth that could sink Dr. Davis's tolerance with just a few choice sentences. Armed with my honesty, there was no telling what damage I could do; I might even alienate the doctor, whom Scott had grown to respect and trust for having sustained my life all these post-transplant years. Scott scheduled an office visit for me—for us—so that he might have some control over my irreverence and lawlessness; I was going to break rules.

"Please come in, Amy." Dr. Davis had already turned and begun walking away from me before finishing this invitation. He set off in those swift giant steps of his. I tried to keep up.

"Um, Scott is on his way. He's in traffic," I blurted out, a bit breathless and still a few Davis-size paces behind him.

"Then let's begin and Scott can join us when he arrives," he called back to me over his shoulder, then made a sharp left and disappeared into his office. I jogged the last few feet to catch up.

"How are you feeling?" he said. This was rote; he always began this way, not only with me but with secretaries and assistants I'd seen him pass by in the hallway, without slowing his step to wait for an answer. This empty question rolled off his tongue so mechanically, and with such lack of interest, I'd always felt justified in ignoring it.

"I don't want to suffer anymore," I said.

It was his turn to ignore me. Out came the patient information form, as if from nowhere, and Dr. Davis launched into the same list of questions, in the same order and the same detached monotone as always. The reason for my visit with him almost didn't matter; the format was most important. Today especially I had the impression that this structure—frustrating as it was for me as the patient—gave Dr. Davis a feeling of being grounded in the face of nebulous transplant complaints like "suffering." Even before he broke into a dull recitation of the checklist, I had already run through the questions in my mind and knew that, based on them—plus a quick blood-pressure check and a perfunctory listen to my heart—it would appear that I was in fine transplant health. Dr. Davis's form of inquiry was inherently flawed.

"Trouble sleeping? Troubles with vision? Ears okay? Sore throat? Dizziness, fainting? Weakness in arms or legs? Nose bleeds? Palpitations? Difficulty urinating? Bowels okay? Cough? Bringing up any phlegm? Headaches? Chest pain? Shortness of breath? Shortness of breath lying down?"

I said *no* to each of these in turn and then anticipated the final two questions, which were the only ones I would not be able to answer with a simple yes or no.

"Appetite?"

This was a loaded question for many heart-transplant patients who were plagued by irresistible food cravings that supposedly accompany high doses of prednisone. Dr. Davis was famous among gossipers in the transplant clinic for his disdain for patients who packed on the pounds. The appetite inquiry was unnecessary for me; I'd never gained weight after my transplant, not even with the hunger pangs of steroids, and he knew it.

I told him my appetite was fine.

"Mood?" he asked. Dr. Davis always saved this one for last. Even though it wasn't a question that could be answered with a simple yes or no, I knew he would be looking for a one-word reply, like *good* or *lousy*. He could jot this down on the paper in front of him in a split second and put an end to the question-and-answer period, which seemed to be his least favorite part of the exam (all that human interaction, you know). Then we'd move on to the blood-pressure cuff at true Davis speed, and before I knew it I'd be walking out the door. But he and I both knew this was not how things were going to progress today.

The mood question was the perfect place to begin. It might have appeared that I had already answered it when I replied to his earlier question about how I was "feeling." He understood what it meant for me to say that I didn't want to suffer anymore; a heart-transplant patient who refused to endure a steady stream of health problems was someone who simply could not live for very long, someone who could not be saved by the best efforts of her doctor. Living sick is an unavoidable part of heart transplantation, and although Dr. Davis tried in earnest to make things more tolerable for his patients ("We need to get you feeling well again," he'd said to me repeatedly over the years), he simply could not do it; his hands were tied by the ropes of immunosuppression. Never free to advise his patients to abandon their medications, he was bound to cause them perpetual anguish even as he sustained their tenuous lives. There was just no saving heart-transplant patients without harming them as well.

Maybe that's where Dr. Davis's scowl came from. I imagined that the reality of transplant was not easy for him to face as he slipped into his long white coat each morning. Could it have caught him up in some kind of psychological whirlwind; perhaps along the lines of the one I found myself in today as I sat in his office? I'd been spinning in this theory for seventeen years—Dr. Davis had to have been at it for even longer—and over this time I'd come to identify this seeming vortex by name: the *mind fuck* of heart transplantation.

"How do you think my mood is, Dr. Davis?" It was the first time I'd ever answered one of his questions with one of my own.

Silence.

"I had a sore throat that turned into lymph node surgery! How does that sound to you?"

"So I heard. I'm sorry."

There was no apology in his eyes.

"No, *I'm* sorry! I'm sorry I had my armpit sliced open for no good reason. In case you don't know, the whole thing was unnecessary. The surgeon pretty much told me so when she felt the lump in the first place. She told me it felt like *nothing;* she wouldn't even pay attention to it in a normal patient. But she couldn't take any chances because I'm a transplant patient—destined to die from some terrible cancer at any moment, right? Cover your ass, doctor, there's a heart-transplant girl in the room! You know the drill." I paused to see what effect, if any, my sassiness had on him. None, apparently. I took this apparent indifference as permission to continue. "I consulted with an oncologist too, and he agreed with the surgeon—the size and shape of the lump didn't seem particularly worrisome—but in a transplant body, who knows? It was the same scared bullshit all over again. I tried to pull some reasoning out of him. I mean, wouldn't it be strange for me to get lymphoma now, after seventeen years on this medicine? He told me no, one of his lymphoma patients had a heart transplant sixteen years ago. Oh, great! Two doctors were telling me I didn't really need surgery but I had to have it anyway. Yeah, sure, that makes lots of sense! It was a total mind fuck."

There. I'd done it. Cursed in front of Dr. Davis. Threw my lewd metaphor right in his face.

He didn't flinch.

"The man with the lymphoma is my patient too," he said. "Yes, he is sixteen years out, but he is not you. He's had trouble with artery disease for a long time now, and I've had to keep his immunosuppression very high. It's probably what led to the cancer. But I wouldn't expect to see lymphoma show up in you at this point. At your level of medicine, it would be most unlikely."

"So the surgery was unnecessary," I said.

"I guess so. Maybe. I'm sorry."

Dr. Davis would become more certain of it later on, during the physical examination part of the appointment, when he would confirm once and for all that the rush to surgery had indeed been baseless and terribly unfortunate. He reached under my right arm—the one that had not been operated on—and found a lump similar in size and shape to the corresponding one that had been removed from my other armpit. "If I'd felt that, I never would have sent you for surgery," he said.

But of course he hadn't, because he hadn't been there. Dr. Davis might have saved me from an awful surgery and prevented needless torment with just one phone call from California—maybe telling the oncologist to hold off because lymphoma was less likely in me than in my sixteen-year post-transplant peer. Or he could have chosen to call me directly—perhaps ask me to check under my other arm and make a comparison of nodes. Dr. Davis could have put out the fire of urgency and the rush to surgery, if nothing else. But he didn't. He failed me. Let me down when I really needed him. The unnecessary surgery was all his fault.

I readied myself to throw the first punch.

"I wish you'd been here," I said. It was more a love tap than a right hook.

The venom just wouldn't come—and I needed it now. Time was running out; Scott would arrive any minute, and then I'd have to pull back from anger and watch my mouth. But I found myself strangely unable to lash out at Dr. Davis in the way I'd intended. There wasn't any fervor in it anymore. When it came down to it, I doubted my own rage. All at once I felt unjustified in my expectations. Dr. Davis was, after all, only my doctor. He'd never really been Ron to me, had he? And maybe I'd never been his favorite patient. Why should he call me during his vacation when he could just send an e-mail to my transplant nurse? Why should he deal with the lump under my arm when he could send me off to a specialist? I was too seasoned a patient to allow myself to balk at what was really just a typical doctor handoff, the same kind of punt I'd seen dozens of times. To unleash my anger at Dr. Davis would be like clobbering him for not loving me enough. Who said he had to love me at all? Heart-transplant doctors don't even have to care about their patients, let alone love them; all they have to do is try to keep them alive as long as possible. At seventeen years post-transplant, I was living proof that Dr. Davis had fulfilled his obligation to me and then some.

"I'm sorry," he said. "I was away on vacation when it happened."

"Well, you're here now," I said, "and I can tell you, I'm completely unraveled. For one thing, I can't even move my left arm—"

"That will come back. The nerves will regener—"

"It's not just the arm, Dr. Davis. It's the years of crap just like this. It's illness and hospitals and specialists and denervated heartbeats and immunosuppression. I don't want to do it anymore. The lymphoma is just the last straw."

"You don't have lymphoma. The preliminary labs look fine."

"Right. So it's on to the next illness, the next infection, the next cancer scare, the next heart biopsy—and I'm going to feel sick the whole time. There's no end, and you know it."

He didn't disagree.

"No, wait. Actually there is an end. It ends when I die. And I've been thinking a lot about dying lately, Dr. Davis. It's a real option for me." The words were coming fast and loud. "I've been working my ass off in this body, spinning my wheels all these years, and it's gotten me nowhere—except to this lymph node surgery and to new kinds of pain that I'd never imagined. I think I deserve a rest, don't you?"

He didn't. By Hippocratic oath, he couldn't.

"We need to get you feeling well again," he said.

"You always say that. It's pure bullshit!"

Scott walked into the office at that moment and stopped dead. He dropped down into the chair beside me, mouth agape. I continued on, undaunted. "I've been waiting to feel well for seventeen years. Why should it be possible now? Don't hold out false hope to me. I've been at this too long. I'm too smart. Please, please, just tell me something that isn't a lie."

I was yelling now. Scott was lit with reproach.

"Dr. Davis is only trying to help, Amy." I could feel Scott's eyes on me when he said this, but I dared not turn my head to face him. Instead, I shifted my line of vision down and to the side. I could see his hands, which were gripping the side of the chair like a safety bar on a roller coaster. *Stop acting like a child and alienating your doctor—right now!* his hands said to me, shaking and blood red from the squeezing.

"We need to make it so you can do the things that are important to you—things that make you feel like *you*," Dr. Davis said.

"Oh, please, you can't be serious. I haven't been me for seventeen years. Amy is gone. I'm just a sick girl." I paused, sensing that my talking time should have been up by now. But Dr. Davis was staying put, allowing me to go on. "You didn't know me before I got sick. I wasn't like this."

Before I got sick. I hardly remembered what life was like in a healthy body; memories of pre-transplant Amy appeared vaguely in my mind like childhood fables and bedtime stories from a lifetime ago. There were only photos to remind me of what used to be; one in particular would make me cry every time I looked at it: the photo of me standing in front of a lake in my striped bikini. I had my arms stretched way out to the sides, my head thrown back, mouth open wide, and I was laughing. It was a sunny day and everything was trouble-free. I was twenty-four years old and in love.

Scott wouldn't let go of the camera that afternoon. He kept taking pictures of me, one after the other, as if I were a swimsuit model. He couldn't get enough. I remembered telling him not to use the whole roll of film just on me, and he'd made some joke about how he wanted all the photos he could get, just in case I decided to up and leave him forever.

I sure was pretty once, wasn't I? And carefree. I'd had my own heart back then, and my spirit. I was joyful and giddy and full of hope. I didn't know what death felt like. I had innocent eyes—like everyone else I knew.

"What gives your life meaning, Amy?" I'd lost myself in thought for a moment, and now Dr. Davis was bringing me back. I wasn't sure if he was serious or not; *meaning* had never been on his list of questions before. As if he'd prepared in advance for this discussion, Dr. Davis began rattling off possibilities for me, beginning with the most obvious: "There's Scott and Casey, maybe the law—"

"I don't want to practice law."

"And then there's your family—your father—"

He'd put me in a tight spot here. Wives were supposed to find life-sustaining meaning in their relationships with their husbands, at least if the marriage was a good one. And mothers were always supposed to find meaning in their children; I'd be a bad mother if I were to say I was not willing to keep myself alive for the sake of my son. I knew there would be no escape from condemnation for what I was about to say.

"I love my family, but I can't live for them. Maybe that makes me a bad person, I don't know. But Scott gets up every morning and goes to work, and my son goes to school. And I'm at home feeling sick. Or at the hospital. I can't just be this fixture that hangs around so the people I love can check in on me every now and then while they go along with their busy lives. Call me selfish, but I need to have some meaning besides living only for other people."

Dr. Davis looked stumped. His jaw slackened and his mouth fell open a bit. He hadn't expected me to answer this way.

For a few seconds, no one spoke.

I slumped down in my chair. Sure, my life had meaning and I knew just what it was. Dr. Davis should have known as well. More than anything else, the meaning of my life was survival. It had to be. How could I get to other things if I weren't alive? Survival was the first thing on my mind when I got up each morning. It was the prerequisite to everything else that could possibly be important in my life. For me, any meaning that was not connected to staying alive was a luxury, a frivolous nonnecessity, a fantasy. It would take my most dedicated imagination to answer Dr. Davis's question today. I would have to do the unthinkable: put my heart transplant aside and dream.

"I'd like to write."

Dr. Davis perked up immediately. "Why not write, then?"

"I've tried. I've even enrolled in writing classes a couple of times, but then I got sick and missed most of the semester."

Scott chimed in. "You don't need a class. Just sit down and write. You're a great writer." I knew he meant this as encouragement, but all I could hear was invalidation.

"I used to be a writer—when I wasn't a sick girl. I haven't written anything since college. I'd need a class or something to help me get going again."

"No, you wouldn't. That's just an excuse. Maybe you just don't really want to do it," Scott said.

I turned my head away from this remark and focused on Dr. Davis again. He'd become more of an ally than Scott over the last five minutes. "If I could write a book—or maybe even books—if I could live long enough to do it, that would have meaning for me."

"Then that's what you should do!" Dr. Davis rang out, his eyes wide with an uncharacteristic sparkle as if he'd just discovered something rare and wonderful. The corners of his lips curled up into a smile that was so unfamiliar it made me feel more than a little bit embarrassed. I pulled back from his creepy enthusiasm.

Wait a minute. What was going on here? What happened to my appointment with Dr. Davis today, the meeting that was supposed to be a showdown? Who was this imposter grinning at me from across the desk? What happened to the doctor who hadn't strayed from his list of questions in seventeen years? I didn't come here to ponder the meaning in my life; I'd come to tell Dr. Davis that he'd failed me. It was the day I would tell it to him straight.

"If I can't be well, I don't want to live anymore."

This was, of course, suicide talk. Scott covered his eyes with his hands when I said it. Dr. Davis lost his smile. Meaning flew out the window. But I didn't mind; I'd regained control over my doctor's appointment. For a minute there, it had almost gotten away from me, turned into a pep rally for hopes and dreams when I'd meant for it to be a final good-bye.

"I'm going to stop taking my medicines—all of them. And then you can see, Dr. Davis; you can see what happens to someone who's seventeen years out when they stop the poison. Maybe I'll live, maybe not. I can be an experiment."

Kaboom! I'd blown everything to bits—obliterated my perfect-patient image and killed off any pride Dr. Davis might have taken in helping me stay alive for so long. I'd abandoned ship, gone AWOL, left the battle scene of my heart-transplant life in utter disgrace. Had I no regard for the mission of my dedicated captain, my leader? My longevity had always been Dr. Davis's task, beating the odds, accumulating post-transplant years like Medals of Honor. And with each annual exam, he'd claimed a successive victory—for us. Now, though, it seemed Dr. Davis and I had arrived at the point where we were fighting for different things. It felt to me like we weren't on the same side anymore.

"Let's lower your medicines," he said, light as a breeze.

"You can't be serious."

"I think we can lower them and you'll be fine. You can start tomorrow and then check your blood levels in two weeks."

"How is that possible?"

"It's fine," he said, reverting back to his old self again—a dismissive doctor who wasn't up for a whole lot of discussion. I realized for the first time that I actually liked him better this way.

"I'll think about it," I said, unable to surrender just yet. Only a minute ago, this guy had been the enemy.

"I want to see you again next week so we can talk. And I'd like to see you once a week for a while—until you're feeling . . . better. More yourself." He rose to his feet and nodded quick and sharp, like a salute without hands. This meeting was now over.

Scott and I followed his lead to the door. Dr. Davis lingered there for a moment with his hand on the knob.

"Oh, and Amy . . . if you like, I can contact someone at the university about arranging for a writing tutorial with a professor there. You could do things on your own schedule. Might make it easier."

I told him I'd have to think about that too.

I was caught up in olive branches.

29

We stood waiting for the elevator like strangers. Scott positioned himself in front of the bulletin board by the far wall. I remained opposite him, over by the glass case that held a directory of the fifth-floor doctors, their names in little plastic letters, alphabetized and pressed into horizontal grooves in dusty brown felt. About twenty names were listed; I counted them, just to distract myself, and then began to add up how many of them belonged to specialists who'd had a crack at solving some inscrutable ill presented to them by my transplant body at one time or another. I reached nine in my tally before the elevator arrived.

I half expected Scott to wait for the next one so we wouldn't have to ride down together in a small square box. I could tell a storm was brooding in him by the way he stuffed his hands deep into his pockets and forced a fake, tuneless whistle from his lips. Scott was not a whistler. And always after leaving a doctor's appointment with me, one of his hands would find mine long before we'd reached the elevator. We would move through the hospital lobby in perfect step, stride matching stride, one of those couples entwined so seamlessly as to appear nearly continuous. Then there would be a lengthy hug once we cleared the building, and sometimes a lingering kiss as well—especially when the medical news of the day had been good.

But today there had been no news for us to judge, good or bad: only consequences, and these arose almost instantaneously from a strained conversation between doctor and patient. The aftershocks were already there to see and feel. Scott and I stood divided from each other today. We rode the elevator down in silence, retreating to safe corners in the far back so that a neutralizing cluster of unfamiliar faces and bodies could come between us until we reached the lobby.

The elevator doors opened and the buffer disappeared. We were the last to step out: Scott quickly, me lingering.

"See you at home," he said. Scott was headed for his car. He brushed past me, lifting his hand up in a sweeping motion that was half *Good-bye, see you later,* and half *would you just get out of here?*

"You're mad at me." I stopped walking, planted my feet in defiance, chest out, hands in tight fists down by my sides, and called out from a few paces behind. "You're actually mad at me!"

Scott paused beside the revolving door of the lobby and looked down at the scuffed tile floor as if it were the saddest thing he'd ever seen. "I don't know what I am right now. I really don't."

Two confident strides forward, and I came to a stop just inches below Scott's chin, stubbornly determined to make my case before I lost him to the maze of a busy parking lot. "You should be mad at Dr. Davis, not at me."

"I don't want to talk about this. Not here."

I plowed on. "So now he tells me I can lower my medicine level! Great, after I've been begging him to do it for ten whole years. And Dr. Wonderful, he's going to help get me a writing professor? It's like he's turned into the Easter Bunny or something. But you know, Davis is just grabbing at the air. The man is fresh out of ideas. He can't save me from this ridiculous body—"

"Of course he can't. No one can save you. It's not fair to expect Dr. Davis to make everything okay. You had a heart transplant. It's been seventeen years. What do you expect? *You have a transplanted heart, Amy.*"

Scott had never said this to me before. Neither one of us had ever stated the truth this way—out loud and so starkly. Heart transplant had not been a state of being that defined me. It was simply background for our life together. We took it as a given and then did our best to rise above the challenges and hold on to the things that my heart should have taken away from us. Sometimes we felt close to succeeding.

Never more close then when we'd go hiking up mountains. It was an unlikely activity for a couple like us; Scott had never even hiked before we met, and I wasn't particularly interested in scaling peaks before my transplant. But from our first hill walk together, Scott and I noticed the incomparable feeling we'd get from completing an ascent together—standing at the top and marveling at our accomplishment. There, at the crest of our effort, we triumphed in having done the difficult—or, later, atop taller mountains, the nearly impossible—in spite of a challenging heart. Hiking high and long would become a way to surmount all the bad things that were supposed to hold us back. And so began our love for mountains—and for climbing them together.

There I'd be, alongside Scott, perched on a ledge after hiking for hours, up, up, up, beginning at a high-altitude point and then climbing into even thinner air that made us gasp—both of us—and laugh at our breathlessness. Again, my heart transplant was there with us on that ascent, but only in a way that lifted our spirits; we would think of it with silent pride when passing fellow trekkers who got tuckered out and turned back down the mountain. Forging on past them, we would arrive finally at a panoramic vista and find ourselves alone—the climbers who had persisted beyond all expectation—basking in a moment of silent recognition of the true obstacle overcome. As I looked out over the blue-green treetops below, the lakes and valleys, and the rocky ledges we'd scaled with hands and feet and grit, I felt a surge of giddy pride. *Look what you've done, Amy. You climbed a mountain—with a transplanted heart in your chest. That's some crazy kind of amazing.*

Then it would be time for a scenic photo. On one of our hikes in the Tetons, I took the camera from my backpack and told Scott to stand over by the wooden sign that marked the altitude on that spot: 6,000 feet. I didn't have to ask him to smile. High above the world, above the heart transplant of his beloved wife, Scott stood proud and free with his hands firmly on his hips, elbows out to the side, puffed like a peacock. Well past the point of his greatest hopes—the dreams he dared not dream.

Purely happy.

I took the picture.

Freeze time. Freeze time. Freeze time. That's what we'd say to each other at times like this in a moment of freedom from heart-transplant troubles. We'd huddle together nose against nose and repeat it to each other in breathy unison, part mantra, part desperate plea: *Freeze time, freeze time. . . .* But today, as Scott stood slumped in front of that revolving hospital door, there didn't feel like much left to freeze anymore. The denervated heartbeats of a twenty-five-year-old girl had matured into those of a forty-two-year-old woman and were increasingly complicated and difficult to abide.

"I said I don't want to talk about this now," he said.

"Okay. But you're wrong about Dr. Davis. He wasn't there when I needed him."

"That may be. But it doesn't give you the right to do what you did in that appointment today. No illness gives you that right. The way you acted and the things you said to him about stopping your medicine were so . . . beneath you."

"Sorry, but under the circumstances, there's not a whole lot that's *beneath* me. What you saw today in Davis's office is the best I can do right now."

"No, it isn't; don't tell me that. I think you can do better." Scott was calm, so sure of himself in this moment that he sounded almost matter-of-fact.

I didn't know whether to laugh or throw a punch. "How can I do better? You tell me how."

"You know how. It's all up to you. It's in your hands, and you know it."

Here it was again: the moment of choice. It had been there in front of me before, in the silence that hung in the air after my desperate father had just finished begging me *please* to say yes to the heart transplant. It had been there in the enduring instant when Scott slipped a wedding ring on my finger and I vowed beneath my veil never to take him for granted or let my heart transplant get in the way of our love. I'd heard this great moment of choice ring out in the first cry of a baby—my baby—in the middle of the night, as the sound pushed aside my replacement heart and moved to the forefront a new life more important than my own. And it had been there again in the pause on a mountain trail when I decided between turning around and pushing forward.

Scott wanted me to reach deep down and pull out the strength he knew was still there. That was how I could do better than I'd done today in Dr. Davis's office: by putting the sick girl aside—even if just for a moment—and summoning the Amy who was buried underneath. Every once in a while, necessity would come along and call her out of the rubble heap—make her come up for air, show her pretty face again, and her indomitable will. Because her life depended on it.

The call had come again.

"Find that strength of yours. You know it's in there," Scott said finally, beaming with an intensity that pierced straight through me.

"I'll try."

He pushed through the revolving door. As it made the half turn I noticed a hint of a smile, a softening in the tight line that had become Scott's lips. His Amy never tried to do something. She just did it.

Post-Game

My family has returned from the Super Bowl. With suitcases full of laundry.

Now there is a pile of dirty clothes in front of my basement door. I look down at it, pressing the curve of a plastic basket against my hip. This is going to be at least four loads. How can two people make so much laundry over just one weekend?

"Check out my new hat, Mom!" Across the room, Casey holds up his Super Bowl cap and waves it in the air.

"What hat? I can't see from here. Come show me."

He jogs over to where I am standing. "This hat," he says. "It's the coolest one ever. See this brown stuff here?" He points to the beige woven material on the front. It is a special cap.

"Doesn't it look great on me?" he says.

I reach down and grab one of Scott's T-shirts from the pile on the floor and toss it on top of his head. "I think this looks even better!"

"Hey!" he says, giggling, pulling it off and throwing it back my way, along with a pair of underpants snagged with it. And then he is off, running somewhere. Always running, that boy of mine.

I set the basket down on the floor and begin to separate white socks from dark pants. On my knees, sorting through the mound of damp, dirty clothing, I piece together a few moments from the father-son weekend by the food stains and small bits of dirt and gravel that I find. There was something barbecued, perhaps. There was a Popsicle. Someone fell in the grass, maybe. I will never know for sure. I was not there.

I was here—sorting through my life. Looking for reasons to put medicine in my mouth, and finding enough of them to be able to swallow.

Scott walks over and stands above me. He is smiling. "We really had a lot of fun," he says.

"I'm so glad," I say, throwing the last sock into the white pile. He reaches down and helps me up from the floor. Without letting go, he slides his hands up my arms and around to my back, pulling me into an embrace. His shirt collar smells like the inside of an airplane. I realize for the first time how far away he has been this weekend.

"You smell like everything wonderful," he says, nuzzling into my neck. I pull him closer and lift the heels of my hands off his back. Then with my fingers splayed out like starfish, I begin to press the flat centers of my palms against his rib cage.

Does he realize I'm about to breathe him in?

He may never know the things I have taken from him in this way, with my hands pressed to his body. Like the laundry basket filled with clues, the Amy in his arms contains only hints of the full story. How much can we really know for sure anyway, beyond our own selves?

Not very much, I've come to realize, through the skewed wisdom of illness.

And yet I still long for Scott to know me in a way that might be impossible. Wrapped in his arms at this moment, I want him to recognize that my heart-transplant sadness does not mean he has failed to make me happy. Nor does it mean I don't adore him.

Through the soft creases of my palms, I begin to inhale now. There is warmth, a tingling. A sense that everything is okay. It is the feeling of my Scotty. He fills me with his air and I float away, easy, like a balloon into the sky.

I pat Scott on the rear end and send his jet-lagged body upstairs. *You go grab a shower and relax. I'll finish cleaning up down here.* There is still so much I want to tell him—about the limitations of this sick girl and the expansiveness of her love.

I will begin with the white load.

IN GRATITUDE

I AM GRATEFUL TO THE PEOPLE WHO KEPT ME MOVING FORWARD IN writing this book—despite the self-doubts of a first-time writer and regardless of the creeping discomfort that comes with putting one's life on paper.

My most sincere thanks to:

My steadfast transplant cardiologist who has been by my side and in my heart—in spirit and in fact—through twenty years of hairpin turns and death-defying acts.

Lenny Stern, my earliest champion and first reader, who urged me on with just the right mixture of humor, praise, critical wisdom, and genuine eagerness.

Stephen Koch, teacher and mentor from the start, who freed me to put pen to paper in the first place and to confront the empty page courageously until my job was done.

The birthday group girls, my dearest friends and biggest fans—Lauren Stern, Deirdre Cohen, Jane Kimmel, and Jill Dresner —ever complimentary as I dipped my toe into the uncertain waters of writing—such wonderful friends who possess the love, the willingness to listen, and the bravery to remind me of who I am when illness makes it all too easy to forget.

So many good friends who keep me laughing, thinking, and learning: my sister, Jodie Hirsch, Leslie Hinderstein, Sue Resnick, Valerie Yellin, Joy Cianci, Ann Silverstein, Jola Skandunaite, Tony Contorno, and Jen Cook.

My father and step-mother, Arthur and Beverly Shorin, who have grown in strength and understanding along with me over the years, especially as I began to put their experiences and mine into writing. I couldn't ask for better allies, friends, and parents.

Rebecca Gradinger, my remarkable agent at Janklow and Nesbit, an ardent supporter who swept me up and away on an amazing ride that has been the publishing of this book. So talented and unrelenting in her efforts, navigating the journey always with a sense of calm and insight, Rebecca has worked wonders for this book and for me as a writer.

Elisabeth Schmitz at Grove Atlantic, my brilliant editor who grasped every nuance of this complex story from the start and helped distill my writing down to its very best elements. Having Elisabeth as my first editor—a joyous experience from beginning to end—I feel most fortunate and fear I may have been spoiled for the rest of my writing life.

AFTERWORD

As I place my fingers on the keyboard, Scott is on a plane on his way home from the Super Bowl.

Three years after he returned home from a different Super Bowl trip and deposited a pile of dirty clothes by the basement door, I find myself back where my book began—with me at a laptop, taking a deep breath as I unzip my life in front of the stark white screen. With a small gasp, I realize that it is things like seasonal football games and laundry heaps that are the most exquisite markers of existence and time. They are signs of the ongoing, the sturdy recurrence of the mundane that, when you stop to look at it, is extraordinary.

At least it is to me.

I am alive at twenty years post heart transplant. Hike, pass, catch. Wash, dry, fold. My life goes on, as routine as it is miraculous.

Yet here is my book—a memoir—that removes the mask from the miracle, that peels away the illusion of normalcy in my post-transplant life. Fantastic science and a wondrously donated heart may have saved my life, but there is nothing fantastic or wondrous about living sick and scared since the age of twenty-four. And herein lies the conflict: I can pause mid-sentence, misty with appreciation for my astounding good fortune in being alive, and at the same time proclaim how tough it is to live in a heart transplant body. The duality has become second nature to me over time. But to others, the flip side to a miracle has been a surprise.

"The book stunned me. Couldn't put it down, I tell you. What you've said here is completely new—and important," a writer for *U.S. News and World Report* told me on the phone. True surgical success, he realized more than ever, is more than just avoiding infections and medical mishaps after all. People need to know what happens *after* a lifesaving heart transplant—after the cameras turn away from the medical triumph and a patient is left to live the aftermath of chronic illness and a brand new fight for survival. He couldn't wait to write about it in his column.

Why is it that something as complicated and dramatic as a heart transplant has been seen as simply a miracle when so few things in life, if any, are so clear cut? Has it been just too unsettling to consider the possibility that an awe-inspiring, lifesaving surgery might be a mixed bag?

I received a new heart and am still here twenty years later, yes. Scratch the surface, though, and a different side of my longevity emerges. Every day I fight hard to keep this heart going.

There are people who would prefer I kept my reality hidden. One reader wrote, "Amy dear, take your medicine and shut up."

I pause for a moment, exhale, and remember something a friend said when I forwarded her a copy of that reaction, "You know what we should do? Let's lift his little comment and put it onto T-shirts we can all wear!"

By "all" she meant the administrators, nurses, doctors, and kids at her workplace—a haven for sick children, many of them chronically ill. My friend knows well the poisonous effect that the command "shut up" can have on those who live with incurable illness. To emblazon the censorious decree across our chests would explode its cruelty, fly in the face of the mandate that we must always wear the mask and preserve the illusion.

I am inspired to take the T-shirt suggestion and run with it—at least in my imagination; break away from these paragraphs and head upstairs, grab one of Scott's undershirts and a couple of fat

Magic Markers, and write that reader's mandate in big letters across the front. Then, turning the shirt over, I switch markers from black to bright blue and scrawl something else.

Go Giants!

Freed by this image, I am at once filled with renewed confidence that there is no shame in being honest about the flip side. Envisioning my head and arms poking through an inked-up white T-shirt, I arrive at an end to my book that speaks as loud as its beginning: there is nothing simple about my heart transplant life. Despair most certainly can coexist with joy. Anger with hope. Sadness with gratitude.

Tears with cheers.

A GROVE PRESS READING GROUP GUIDE
BY BARBARA PUTNAM

Sick Girl

Amy Silverstein

ABOUT THIS GUIDE

We hope that these discussion questions will enhance your reading group's exploration of Amy Silverstein's *Sick Girl*. They are meant to stimulate discussion, offer new viewpoints, and enrich your enjoyment of the book.

More reading group guides and additional information, including summaries, author tours, and author sites for other fine Grove Press titles, may be found on our Web site, www.groveatlantic.com.

QUESTIONS FOR DISCUSSION

1. Throughout the book Amy seeks to find her identity and protect it. What are the ways she establishes who she is? What are some of the assaults to her view of herself? How does illness inexorably set her apart? (Think about times people avert their eyes, isolating her. Her parents? A phalanx of residents around her bed? Even doctors whose expertise she threatens?) "This doctor couldn't possibly be angry with me because I, Amy—the law student, the young woman, the whole person—wasn't there anymore. His blank stare told me so" (p. 80). Imagine Amy's speaking of "her diluted self" (p. 81) even before the transplant operation.

2. Describe Scott from the heady days of early courtship through the years of struggle and triumph. He is in many ways extraordinary, not only in his own achievements, but also in his almost unbelievable devotion to Amy at every crisis, every test. How does his dedication give us a measure of the woman he loves?

3. When is Amy faced with her biggest challenges? When is she absolutely flattened and ready to give up? Is the reader able to empathize with her despair based on her honest account? Who and what save her?

4. "Sick girl." When and how is the label first stuck on Amy? (p. 70). How does she respond to the term? Is she delimited or rather challenged by the words? Has she chosen an apt, if provocative, title for her memoir?

5. Do you think Amy is "an ungrateful patient" (p. 73) as she herself sometimes worries? How do you react to her lambasting her doctors? Refusing to offer her heart as Exhibit A to the student doctors in Philadelphia? How does Scott try to protect her from her violent reactions?

6. Talk about Amy's relationships with her doctors. How do her attitudes evolve? (p. 223). Yet, as in other aspects of her health and life, just when she thinks she has a handle on something, it shifts. Good news morphs into bad or ambiguous (p. 241). Does she ask for unrealistic support from her doctors? Are their own reservations about friendship reasonable? When we are ill, are we driven to consider our doctors infallible? "There were doctors who were supposed to know it all but who knew only enough about heart transplants to recognize that I presented a challenge beyond their comfort level . . . With a patient like you, it's hard to be sure about anything" (p. 245). And the longer Amy survives, the more it is uncharted territory for everyone. Who are the doctors who stand out as humane individuals?

7. Is it normal that Amy is bitter about her childhood? What was her mother like? Having been ignored and exploited from the age of five on, is it another measure of her determination that she refuses to let that bitterness poison the rest of her life? How does the same strength of character reveal itself in her illness?

8. Amy takes enormous pride in her mothering of Casey (and in Scott's and her parenting together.) Instead of recapitulating her own childhood disaster, what has she decided to accomplish with Casey? Who has been a rich surrogate mother for Amy? Can you recall examples?

9. What does friendship mean to Amy? Scott, of course, is closest and most dependable. Who are other essential friends? How do they support her? What is it about her illness and her pride that complicates relationships?

10. Amy is quick to observe a "self-serving" quality in others—and is often wickedly funny about it. Do you sometimes find a similar trait in Amy? Does her bone honesty compel her to include this less flattering side in her memoir? Is it necessary for her survival that she often needs to be her own cheering squad?

11. A large part of Amy's character is her gratitude. She is generous in her appreciation of many people. Talk about these instances (even if she can sometimes be cranky about the same people.) Her father? Beverly? Her deep gratefulness to Scott is nearly constant. What are some of the many gifts he bestows on Amy, and at what cost? As depicted in her memoir, does Scott emerge nearly as heroic as Amy?

12. How much of the book is Amy's need to reach out? Is a big impetus for the book her need to explain, from behind her loneliness and fear, not only how much she has suffered but also how much she has loved and been loved? Does she succeed in these goals? About Scott, she says, "There is still so much I want to tell him—about the limitations of this sick girl and the expansiveness of her love" (p. 292).

13. Contrast Ellen as a transplant patient with Amy. How does Ellen's smug outsmarting of the doctors' prohibitions differ from Amy's idea of being a "smart patient"? Give examples of Amy's extraordinary discipline, both mental and physical. Does her pushing herself (mountains, Pamplona) sometimes seem

frightening or unwise? Do you think it is this beyond-the-boundaries physical testing that has preserved her?

14. How does Dr. Allen, himself a cancer survivor against dire odds, change Amy's thinking? (p. 256). Is it not only what he says but how he says it? (Contrast him with all the other superstars in operating rooms, too busy to talk to her or hold her hand.) "As long as you live you must fight. Always fight . . . It's not something that begins and ends. You must see it as a journey" (p. 256). What does it mean that he takes both her hands in his, shares his own story and talks to her, unlike other doctors, without science or statistics. "And I was off on my next journey" (p. 257).

15. When are times in the memoir that Amy does not feel like a sick girl? Are they times she can take particular pride in her achievement? Even when she is deceiving others about the ravages of her illness?

16. "If I listened to my heart sounds for too long, I began to imagine them coming together to form a death march" (p. 269). Is it a mark of Amy's ingenuity that she devises a way literally to hug herself for company and comfort?

17. For someone who has always taken pleasure in her body and prettiness, the effects of prednisone and her monumental scar are a test. How does Scott always make her feel like a heroine in a love story, always dazzling in his eyes?

18. What is the essential, terrible paradox of Amy's adult life? "There was just no saving heart-transplant patients without harming them as well" (p. 176). Amy rightly sees her medicines as poisons. "What had once been an integral and vibrant